"WHO IS NURSING THEM? IT IS US."

Neoliberalism, HIV/AIDS, and the Occupational Health and Safety of South African Public Sector Nurses

Jennifer Zelnick

Salem State College
School of Social Work

Work, Health, and Environment Series
Series Editors: **Charles Levenstein, Robert Forrant, and John Wooding**

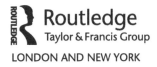

Routledge
Taylor & Francis Group

LONDON AND NEW YORK

First published 2011 by Baywood Publishing Company, Inc.

2 Park Square, Milton Park, Abingdon, Oxon OX14 4RN
711 Third Avenue, New York, NY 10017, USA

Routledge is an imprint of the Taylor & Francis Group, an informa business

First issued in paperback 2017

Library of Congress Catalog Number: 2009046909

ISBN 13: 978-0-89503-327-7 (hbk)

Library of Congress Cataloging-in-Publication Data

Zelnick, Jennifer R., 1964 –
    "Who is nursing them? It is us." : neoliberalism, HIV/AIDS, and the occupational health and safety of South African public sector nurses / Jennifer R. Zelnick.
      p. ; cm. -- (Work, health, and environment series)
    Includes bibliographical references and index.
    ISBN 978-0-89503-327-7 (cloth : alk. paper) 1. AIDS (Disease)--South Africa. 2. AIDS (Disease)--Nursing--South Africa. 3. Neoliberalism. I. Title. II. Title: Neoliberalism, HIV/AIDS, and the occupational health and safety of South African public sector nurses. III. Series: Work, health, and environment series.
    [DNLM: 1. HIV Infections--nursing--South Africa. 2. Acquired Immunodeficiency Syndrome--nursing--South Africa. 3. Nurses--psychology--South Africa. 4. Occupational Health--South Africa. 5. Public Health Nursing--South Africa. WY 153.5 Z51w 2010]
    RA643.86.S6Z45 2010
    362.196'979200968--dc22

                                                                                    2009046909

ISBN 978-0-89503-327-7 (hbk)
ISBN 978-0-415-78439-9 (pbk)

Table of Contents

Preface   v

Acknowledgments vii

Introduction: Understanding a Public Health Crisis from a
   Work Environment Perspective   1

Chapter 1. Globalization and Health in sub-Saharan Africa 17

Chapter 2. Neoliberalism in Postapartheid South Africa and the
   HIV/AIDS Epidemic 33

Chapter 3. The Work Environment of Nurses 49

Chapter 4. Case Study Setting: Three Public Hospitals in
   KwaZulu-Natal, South Africa 63

Chapter 5. Staffing, Occupational Health, and HIV/AIDS 89

Chapter 6. Nurses Speak 129

Chapter 7. Discussion—Breathing Life into Policy: Toward a
   Labor/Work Environment Perspective on a Global Public
   Health Crisis 149

Appendix: Group Interview Results Summary 171

References 175

Index 189

Preface

In the Baywood series *Work, Health and Environment,* the conjunction of topics is deliberate and critical. We begin at the point of production—even in the volumes that address environmental issues—because that is where things get made, workers labor, and raw materials are fashioned into products. It is also where things get stored or moved, analyzed or processed, computerized or tracked. In addition, it is where the folks who do the work are exposed to a growing litany of harmful things or are placed in harm's way. The focus on the point of production provides a framework for understanding the contradictions of the modern political economy.

Despite claims to a post-industrial society, work remains essential to all our lives. While work brings income and meaning, it also brings danger and threats to health. The point of production, where goods and services are produced, is also the source of environmental contamination and pollution. Thus, work, health, and environment are intimately linked.

Work organizations, systems of management, indeed the idea of the "market" itself, have a profound impact on the handling of hazardous materials and processes. The existence or absence of decent and safe work is a key determinant of the health of the individual and the community: what we make goes into the world, sometimes improving it, but too often threatening the environment and the lives of people across the globe.

We began this series to bring together some of the best thinking and research from academics, activists, and professionals, all of whom understand the intersection between work and health and environmental degradation, and all of whom think something should be done to improve the situation.

The works in this series stress the political and social struggles surrounding the fight for safe work and protection of the environment, and the local and global struggle for a sustainable world. The books document the horrors of cotton dust, the appalling and dangerous conditions in the oil industry, the unsafe ways in which toys and sneakers are produced, the struggles to link unions and communities to fight corporate pollution, and the dangers posed by the petrochemical industry, both here and abroad. The books speak directly about the contradictory effects of the point of production for the health of workers, community, and the environment. In all these works, the authors keep the politics front and foremost. What has emerged, as this series has grown, is a body of scholarship uniquely focused and highly integrated around themes and problems absolutely critical to our own and our children's future.

Acknowledgments

I could not have accomplished the original research and manuscript preparation without all those who helped care for Lula and Maeve between 2003-2005: Paul Lyons, Steve Zelnick, Max Lyons, Marilyn and Susan Tobin, Susan Murphy, Arlene and Maria Evans, Amanda O'Donnell, Charmela Moonaman, and the Thompson Street Playgroup; and most especially Deb O'Donnell, Henry O'Donnell, Mary Hardwick, and Alice Monkiewicz. Especially Alice, for help in Florida, at the Cape, in Boston, and New York. Because of this help, I was free from worry since I knew that Lula and Maeve were in loving hands. And thanks to Paul Lyons, my stepdad (1942-2009), who lent me his office, his ear, his example as a teacher, scholar, and person—and most of all his unconditional love and support when I needed it the most.

I thank my dissertation committee, Eduardo Siquiera, Craig Slatin, Ken Geiser, Lenore Azaroff and my chair, Robert Forrant—for thinking that this topic was important and valuable, for their invaluable insight and input, and for caring about a labor/work environment approach to health and the public sector.

Many colleagues in South Africa truly paved the way for me. Without Rajen Naidoo at the Nelson Mandela School of Medicine in Durban, this simply would not have happened. I also thank Thandi Chiliza, Noelle Phillips, Bryan Carpenter, Patrick MacNeill, Laura Campbell, and Honey Allee: for opening your doors. To Nick Henwood and IHRG for the perspective. To Gina and Luka for making Durban home. And to Samantha Willan, for friendship and comradeship.

Without my family, Max, Luisa, Maeve, and Liam O'Donnell there is no way I would have had the perseverance or motivation to complete my research or this manuscript. Thanks for all your love. My husband Max has been a collaborator, instigator, whose views on injustice and disease help to keep me sane.

To all those who participated in interviews—hopefully it makes a difference somewhere down the line. Though I tried to preserve the voices of the nurses and managers who were interviewed for the case study, responsibility for the interpretation is mine alone.

INTRODUCTION

CR EO

Understanding a Public
Health Crisis from a
Work Environment Perspective

On May 1, 2004, union members and staff, health care workers, public health activists, and academics met at 1199 Headquarters in New York City for a conference titled, "Health Care in the Americas: A Right or a Luxury." Sponsored by the World Organization for the Right of People to Health Care, Inc. (WORPHC), it was attended by people from the Americas and Caribbean and conducted in English, French/Creole, and Spanish. Diverse health care systems were represented—from the prized national health care system in Canada, to the highly privatized and technologically advanced system in the United States, and to struggling public health systems in Guyana, Argentina, and the Dominican Republic. Speaker after speaker reported on similar trends: the increasing push toward privatization; the decline in access to health care; the degradation of the health care work environment; the burden on health care workers; and the resistance to these developments mounted by health care workers, their unions, and communities. The message from nurses was particularly clear: poor working conditions related to changes in the health care delivery systems were a serious strain that pushed them toward other work or other countries.

Implicit in the conference agenda was the idea that health care as a right was a critical issue for the people whose job it was to provide that care. The threats to the jobs of health care workers were turning them into advocates for public health. The forces that simultaneously reduced access to health services, robbed people of desperately needed treatments (or put them out of reach), and destroyed the work environments of health care workers, were refocusing health care workers' scope of engagement with the issue of health. In a functioning system, one in which the patient and nurse have most of their needs met, it may perhaps be possible to focus on the physical health of the individual patient in isolation. In the current context, the health of any given patient, sick or well, is inextricably tied to the state of the system that creates the conditions for health and health service provision. The

1

international focus of the May Day conference denoted the second implicit fact: that the forces and issues at hand were global in scope despite their local impacts. The agenda for the New York May Day conference was framed by the impact that globalizing the so-called free market has had on public health. This global framing links the fate of health care workers as they confront work-environment and patient-care issues.

A few months later, at the International AIDS conference in Bangkok, nursing and health care workers figured high on the "Access for All"[1] agenda. The annual AIDS conference is used to focus worldwide media attention on the disease; in 2004, conference coverage and related human interest stories were focused on nursing staff and health services. The human rights advocacy group, Physicians for Human Rights (PHR), used the conference as a platform to unveil an extensive report on the social, economic, and political factors that contribute to "brain drain" of health care workers in the context of the African HIV/AIDS pandemic (PHR, 2004). The report acknowledged that goals of providing treatment cannot be met, even when drugs and funding are available, if skilled health care providers are lacking. As Lincoln Chen, director of Harvard's Global Equity Initiative, writes in the introduction to this report,

> The health worker in the workforce is an old problem with new dimensions. People produce their own health, but their effectiveness depends upon health workers and support systems. Inadequately recognized is that irrespective of money and drugs, health achievements depend upon frontline health workers who connect people and communities to technologies and services. It is the worker who glues together all inputs, such as drugs, vaccines, information, and technologies. Pouring money and drugs at a problem is wasteful if workers are not available, motivated, skilled, and supported. (p. 2)

Dr. Chen goes on to note the reasons for the "precarious" condition of health care work: the neglected state of health systems; the accelerated mobility of the workforce beginning in the latter half of the 1990s; and what he terms the "triple threat" that HIV/AIDS poses to the workforce: increasing the work burden, sickening and killing health care workers, and stigmatizing those who care for people living with HIV/AIDS (PLWA).

The *Boston Globe* reported on a visit during the conference to the Bamrasnaradura Hospital, where a nursing official of the 450-bed Bangkok hospital reported that she had only 200 of 400 nursing slots filled, despite the importance of the hospital to the countries efforts to combat HIV/AIDS (MacGillis, July 23,

---

[1]"Access for All," the title of the XV International AIDS conference held in Bangkok, Thailand, in 2004, referred to the mounting, historic effort to extend antiretroviral treatment (frontline treatment for HIV/AIDS) to the developing world. In 2003, 38 million people were estimated to be living with HIV/AIDS; 25 million of them in Africa (UNAIDS, 2004).

2004). This situation in Southeast Asia is mirrored throughout Africa, where conditions in many countries and regions are even worse.

Both the New York May Day Conference at 1199/SEIU and the far bigger and far more prestigious International AIDS conference in Bangkok, raised and debated issues at the core of this books analysis. How could ARV treatment programs in Africa and other developing countries be "scaled up" without adequate nursing staff? Could national systems be put in place to reach hard-to-access patients facing multiple barriers to treatment? Didn't this kind of public effort fly in the face of privatization and commodification of health care, considered responsible for both the destruction of public health systems and deterioration of working conditions for nurses? How can the brain drain of skilled health care workers from poorer countries be stopped when this defies the logic of policy initiatives such as the WTO general agreement on trade in services and the Bush administration's recent efforts to relax standards for (H1) work visas? Vis-à-vis the global AIDS pandemic, issues such as international labor solidarity, human rights, and commitment to national health programs and public health—often debated in isolation from mainstream large-scale policy dialogue—might emerge in larger policy forums. This is the discourse to which this book can contribute.

Getting to South Africa

My husband, Max O'Donnell, and I did not chose to go to South Africa to learn about public health and infectious disease because of its huge HIV/AIDS epidemic, or the international controversy over the position of its government on HIV/AIDS. We chose South Africa because of its history of social change, the recent overthrow of the apartheid government, and the role of trade unions and the working class in bringing this about. Our perspectives on public health, occupational health in particular, prioritized these events as the most important for the health of the South African people.

As a former union organizer, I was compelled by the question of what was happening within trade unions as South Africa wrestled with the constraints of the global economy and conditions in the region. Knowing that HIV/AIDS affected working-age people, I wondered about the trade union perspective on HIV/AIDS policy. The role of the Congress of South African Trade Unions (COSATU) in the Treatment Action Campaign (TAC), a social movement to fight HIV/AIDS, suggested a powerful public health activist alliance. TAC was led by a Zackie Achmat—cape-colored gay man, former prostitute, and activist in the fight against apartheid—and was assisted by Act-Up and the Treatment Action Group (TAG), very effective U.S./European AIDS activists (Bond, 2005; Epstein, 1996). It partnered with COSATU, the largest and most radical trade union federation in South Africa, and involved growing numbers of poor people living with HIV/AIDS. It seemed that despite the intractable problems associated with the HIV/AIDS epidemic, there would be much to learn from the South African social movement for public health.

In December 2001, Max, our daughter Lula, and I traveled to South Africa for the better part of a year. For my husband (a medical student also pursuing a master's in public health) and I (a doctoral student in work-environment policy), this trip was an opportunity for a break in the midst of studies in order to travel to the epicenter of a historic, tragic disease epidemic; to ground our education in fieldwork in an important part of the world; and to spend time together as a family before our career paths made this more difficult. With a (very) small amount of funding and no clear plan or job waiting for us, we planned a trip to Durban, a seaside, subtropical city on the eastern coast of KwaZulu-Natal, South Africa.

Having chosen our destination, we began to network through public health with South African connections. Through colleagues in Boston, we were fortunate to meet many who played and continue to play a role in South African public health. Dick Clapp of the environmental health program at Boston University, a long time activist in an international group focused on public health in South Africa, introduced us to Leslie London of the Department of Public Health and Primary Health Care at the University of Cape Town, an expert in public/ environmental health and human rights. Jack Geiger, a legendary figure in com-munity health in the United States and South Africa, introduced us to Mervyn Susser and Zena Stein, an extraordinary expatriate South African husband and wife team based at the Mailman School of Public Health at Columbia University.

Through these contacts we forged an understanding of public health and the regional HIV/AIDS epidemic that was grounded in the recent, turbulent, political and social history of KZN. Susser and Stein, both epidemiologists, fled South Africa during the apartheid years, but originally hailed from Durban. They have devoted their lives to researching the determinants of disease for poor South Africans and others, and have been predominant in developing humanistic epidemiology—Susser for exploring how to include levels of causation more appropriate to the social determinants of public health (Schwartz, Susser, & Susser, 1999), and Stein for her long-term commitment and exploration of women's issues, most recently focused on self-protection against HIV/AIDS (Susser, 2002). Susser and Stein were also mentors to so many important scientists, notably Quarraissha and Salim Abdool-Karim, another husband and wife team based in Durban, who write in a 2002 article about the HIV/AIDS epidemic in South Africa (2002):

> The paper is written as a tribute to our mentors Zena Stein and Mervyn Susser, for whom the eighth decade of their lives—the 1990s—was the most challenging of all. Immersed in the struggle against the AIDS epidemic in their native South Africa, they had to bring to bear all of their past experience, and then some. While working with the opposition to the old Apartheid regime, Zena and Mervyn had already anticipated a need for general training

and remodeling in public health after the transition to a democratic society. It soon became clear, however, that history was overturning these plans. As South Africa came under the threat of a catastrophic AIDS epidemic, Zena and Mervyn found their lives largely taken over by a new struggle, the control of HIV/AIDS. By the time of Nelson Mandela's release from prison, it was clear that in the absence of a sustained courageous national intervention, HIV/AIDS was going to have a devastating impact, especially among Black Africans, due to the migrant labour system. Zena and Mervyn were among the first to try to alert the government-in-waiting to the pattern of the epidemic. Their key roles and contributions in the Maputo conference of 1990 remain a testimony to their commitment to the problem of AIDS in South Africa. Since then, and continuing into the present, the largest part of their time has been dedicated to this foremost public health problem of our times, especially training of HIV epidemiologists in South Africa (including the authors). (p. 37)

As a medical student in the 1950s, Jack Geiger, already a civil rights activist in the United States, went to Pholela, South Africa, to work with Sidney Kark at a community-based site that became a model for Community Oriented Primary Care (COPC). A paper by Kark and Cassel (1952) lays out the COPC approach pioneered at the Pholela clinic, and later adopted by the WHO and UNICEF at the 1978 Alma Ata conference. The South African legacy in primary health care is another interesting touchstone for current South African public health research. After realizing the relevance of his South African experience to the U.S. context, Geiger returned to found community health centers in the southern United States and to contribute to the community health movement (Susser, 1999). He maintained ongoing ties and involvement in South Africa, and was an invaluable source of contacts and information for this project.

In 2000 KZN had the highest HIV prevalence in South Africa, estimated to be nearly 37%, based on department of health survey of antenatal clinic data.[2] Durban, the largest city in KZN, played host to the International AIDS conference in 2000, where prominent scientists and public health activists signed a petition that took the African National Congress-led (ANC) government to task for failing to respond to the HIV/AIDS epidemic (The Durban Declaration, 2000). The University of Natal, Durban, and the Nelson Mandela School of Medicine, both located within the city, were historically important in housing opposition groups during the apartheid era and educating minority students. These institutions

---

[2]Estimating the prevalence of HIV is highly problematic in the context where relatively few are actually tested for the disease. Prevalence estimates are based on different data sources, such as household surveys and antenatal clinics. Each type of data presents its own problems with bias and over or under estimation. Updated methods have recently reduced HIV prevalence estimates significantly (UNAIDS, 2007).

employ many who signed the Durban Declaration, including Salim and Quaraissha Abdool-Karim and Hoosen (Jerry) Coovadia.

Quaraissha Abdool-Karim is an epidemiologist and key figure in the national governments initial, well-developed response to HIV/AIDS. Hoosen (Jerry) Coovadia, a pediatrician and the chair of the 2000 Durban AIDS conference, has achieved prominence in international AIDS research. In the spirit of South Africa, they were not only excellent scientists, but committed long-term foes of apartheid, with alliances throughout the country and beyond. People who possess this combination of political activism (with local and international connections) and professional/social contribution are one of the distinguishing characteristics of postapartheid South Africa, providing immensely valuable human capital for social change.

The Research Perspective

In 2002, people living with HIV/AIDS in the United States could expect to live a long and somewhat normal, productive life. This astounding fact was due entirely to the development of antiretroviral (ARV) drug combinations, which included protease inhibitors, a so-called triple cocktail that became widely used in the mid-to-late 1990s. These drugs, developed by U.S.-based pharmaceutical companies, were developed with the support of public research money, which resulted from political pressure from sophisticated activist campaigns led by the Treatment Action Group (TAG) (Irwin, Millen, & Fallows, 2003). ARVs do not cure HIV/AIDS, but turn it into chronic treatable condition like diabetes, and must be taken for a lifetime to manage the condition. ARVs also have historically had a notoriously large price tag; in 2002 the U.S. estimate for a 1-year supply was around $20,000 U.S. (Irwin et al., 2003). The high cost of ARVs meant that these drugs were not available to the vast majority of people living with HIV/AIDS in poorer countries. This appalling differential valuing of human life—a death sentence in one context and a chronic treatable disease in another—is a tragic example of how global inequalities determine health outcomes.

The argument that ARV treatment was too expensive for the world's poor was made in the context of how the world's powerful defined and limited public health. Disability adjusted life years (DALYS) and cost-effectiveness[3] were used to justify the morally baseless argument that certain lives were not worth saving. This approach bases public health decision making on cost-effective

[3] Disability adjusted life years (DALYS) and cost-effectiveness are the cornerstones of the financial approach to health system reform propagated in such documents as the 1993 World Health Report: investing in health (World Bank, 1993). DALYS are a systematic way to measure cost-effectiveness that ascribe monetary value to potential productivity; monetary value is directly related to the potential for economic productivity by an individual in a particular environment.

interventions and the economic worth of lives, and it is related to a set of ideas that translate the ideology of the free market into public policy.

Neoliberal globalization was introduced to sub-Saharan Africa (SSA) through Structural Adjustment Policies (SAPS); this history has been identified as the catalyst for adapting economies in SSA to free-market principals. Of key importance for the situation facing health care workers and the impact of HIV/AIDS is the focus on reducing public spending and encouraging the role of the private sector. While cost is always an important consideration for budgeting public health, placing cost considerations at the center of decision making in health care for the poor, an area that by definition cannot be profitable, skews policies against the least well-off. Further, policies that focused SSA economies on exports that could generate foreign currency profits left a slew of local and national needs unmet, increasing poverty among families and communities. In many countries, the elimination of public funding for health services that took place in an earlier era, along with policies that entrenched new levels of poverty, exacerbated the crisis of HIV/AIDS.

However, Brazil offered an important example of how cost issues could be overcome through a public-sector universal treatment program, even in the context of the general swing toward neoliberal policies. In a 2001 *New York Times Magazine* article, Tina Rosenberg described the program there that provided universal access to ARVs. The public national health program relied on cheaper, generic versions of ARVs (Rosenberg, 2001). The drugs saved lives and also saved vast sums of money through hospitalizations and opportunistic infections prevented. Shortly after this article appeared, a conference hosted by Partners in Health was held at the Harvard School of Public Health on the use of ARVs in "resource-poor settings,"[4] which featured activists, physicians, scientists and politicians from Brazil. Beyond the ARV drugs themselves, the conference focused on a critical issue underlying drugs for treatment: the issue of health care infrastructure for HIV/AIDS treatment. Testing sites and equipment, labs to monitor viral loads and process tests, and properly trained physicians and nurses were some of the basic needs of the treatment programs. Representatives from Brazil stated that "where there is a will, there is a way," claiming that once the political decision to act had been made, everything else would fall into place.

The inroads into the cost of medicines through the use of generics, changed the cost-effectiveness equation sufficiently so that the "high cost of medicines" could reasonably be dispensed with as an argument against treating poor people with

[4]The phrase "resource-poor settings" has become the buzz word for poor countries in the debate over AIDS medicines. It was used in the title of an influential article that came out of Partners in Health at Harvard School of Public Health (Farmer et al., 2001). It is an example of emerging language about HIV/AIDS treatment that bears some rethinking in terms of what it obscures about the dynamics of poverty and underdevelopment.

HIV/AIDS. Generic production revealed the relatively low cost of materials and production of ARVS. So-called high-costs were revealed to actually be patent-protected profits for drug makers, who benefited from public research funding (Irwin et al., 2003). This development appeared to signal a backlash against the application of free-market, neoliberal approaches to international public health.

HIV/AIDS Policy Formation in KZN

Brazil's public HIV/AIDS treatment program benefitted from social movement participation and interplay of a variety of social actors (Berkman, Garcia, Munoz-Laboy, Paira, & Parker, 2005). Thinking about infrastructure in terms of social and human capital led me to undertake research project on HIV/AIDS policy formation at the local and provincial levels in KZN. This 2002 project shaped my understanding of KZN, its health system, and its politics; and allowed me to meet the people who would help me gain entry into three provincial hospitals. This also sparked a desire to return and talk to nurses about their work in the midst of the HIV/AIDS epidemic. From various people with frontline experiences in health care, I learned of the daily struggles of those charged with care and treatment for people living with HIV/AIDS in an environment that offered few supports. Remarks made about the impact of this epidemic on health care workers during a few of my first interviews still ring in my ears.

Salim Abdool-Karim (2002), Chancellor for Research at UND, commented thus in response to a question about HIV/AIDS policy:

> One of the most important things we must do is to show we care about people caring everyday for AIDS patients. We should make anti-retroviral treatment available to these people. Not only because it sets a good example, it's what is needed in this epidemic. We have a very low morale in health care services. Low morale comes from a sense of helplessness to make a difference. People come into health care to make a difference in the world, but all you see are patients dying. (p. 3)

Dr. Patrick McNeil, chief Medical Officer at Port Shepstone district hospital in KwaZulu-Natal described the medical wards on a typical day in 2002, when 60% to 70% of patients were suffering from an AIDS-related illness or were HIV positive (McNeill, 2002). At the time of my interview, Port Shepstone Hospital was initiating a program to prevent the transmission of HIV from mother to child during birth using the drug neviripine.[5] Of 48 volunteers for HIV testing, 41 were

---

[5]This program, called prevention of mother to child transmission (PMTCT) had recently been approved in KZN, despite the fact that it was still opposed by the national government. This was generally recognized as possible for political and personal reasons. KZN is led by a coalition government of the ANC and Inkatha Freedom Party (IFP). The party affiliation (IFP) of the provincial head, and the rumors of HIV impact on his immediate family were reported to have driven this independent policy stance.

found to be positive. Poor morale related to difficulties in providing care was a serious problem described by Dr. McNeill (2002):

> HIV/AIDS patients are time-consuming. They come back, they don't get better, and it is an emotional drain. Young doctors are not trained to see 25-year-olds die, it's not an easy thing to accept. Patients get treated badly— they are in and out 5–6 times with oral thrush and the like. It gets frustrating for the caregivers. These patients are hard to nurse. They must be turned very frequently. We have increased absenteeism among nurses. Some are going for jobs overseas because of the increased stress of nursing HIV+ population. Then there is the issue of occupational exposure through needlesticks. We have 4–5 needlesticks a month, very regularly, and this is quite stressful. Some HIV+ staff are quite sick and are not on anti-retrovirals, and this is another cause of absenteeism. It's a Catch 22. You can't stop it, you are putting out fires. There are a lot of problems with poor nursing of patients, but its not that the nurses are bad. They are overworked, and some are HIV+ themselves. Many are looking after HIV+ relatives, and they will tell you that their cousin, brother, sister have AIDS. It's a huge social disease, with huge impacts beyond just the patients in the hospital.

During a conversation with Sister Zodumo Shange, occupational health nurse at King Edward VIII hospital in Durban, I learned about efforts to encourage nurses to be tested for HIV/AIDS. For the past few years, antiretrovirals had been available in public hospitals for postexposure prophylaxis (PEP) in the event of occupational exposure to HIV/AIDS (KwaZulu-Natal Department of Health, 2001). Post-exposure protocol in the South African public health system is similar to Europe and North America. However, exposed health care workers are required to have an AIDS test prior to administration of ARVs. If the test is positive, prophylaxis is not offered since there is a cost considered by the resource-strapped hospital. Sister Shange reported that without treatment available, and given stigma and questions about the confidentiality of test results at the workplace, most are reluctant to report the needlesticks and obtain prophylactic treatment. She also told me that the situation at King Edward is better than at many hospitals, since King Edward is the site of an ARV pilot project. However, ability to gain access to treatment through this project is limited by eligibility criteria (including responsiveness to the regimen under study) and the fact that study patients are known to the rest of the workforce via their presence at a particular clinic in the hospital. She agreed that post-exposure prophylaxis is a policy that potentially protects health care workers and nurses from becoming HIV positive, but pointed out that context did not support successful implementation of the policy (Shange, 2002).

In South Africa in 2002 development of any policy related to HIV/AIDS was an especially raw, touchy question. In 1990, while in exile, the ANC joined with public health activists at the Maputo conference in Tanzania and produced the Maputo Statement on HIV/AIDS (Stein & Zwi, 1990). The conference resolution recognized "the role that sociopolitical factors, and apartheid specifically, play in facilitating the spread of HIV infection and retarding the control of this epidemic" and that "HIV is not only a medical but a social disease" (p. 142). The Maputo Statement is a radical public health document. It calls for addressing political, social, and economic factors that propel the disease. In particular, it calls political leaders and the ANC to play a vital role:

> Any attempt to deal with the HIV epidemic must be situated within the broader struggle for sociopolitical change. This will provide a context for preventive work amongst the broad group of people most affected by HIV infection. Progressive organizations should inform their membership of the magnitude and importance of HIV infection. They should examine, analyze, and respond to HIV with the support of their membership. We can start by involving senior progressive political leadership within and outside South Africa. The African National Congress (ANC) has a major role to play in this regard. The involvement of political leaders will help overcome suspicion and mistrust created by the South African state. A high public profile will raise awareness and stimulate appropriate action. (p. 137)

When the ANC took office in 1994, one of their first actions was to set up an AIDS directorate staffed by well-known scientists active in the struggle against apartheid (including Coovadia and Abdool-Karim). In 1994 the prevalence of HIV in South Africa was estimated to around 1%; however, by 2000 South African prevalence had reached nearly 23% nationally (Abdool-Karim & Abdool-Karim, 2002). Chris Hani, Spear of the Nation Leader who was assassinated before the ANC took office, predicted this increase.

> Those of us in exile are in the unfortunate situation of being in the areas where the prevalence is high. We cannot afford to allow the AIDS epidemic to ruin the realization of our dreams. Existing statistics indicate that we are still at the beginning of the AIDS epidemic in our country. Unattended, however, this will result in untold damage and suffering by the end of the century-1990. (Abdool-Karim & Abdool-Karim, 2002, p. 38)

The Maputo Statement, Hani's prescience, a politically and scientifically able leadership, and a good organization did not stop the spread of HIV. What followed was a decade of political struggle for the rights of people living with HIV/AIDS and their affected communities. The center of this struggle became the needs of PLWA—needs compounded by high unemployment and cuts in basic services— and the ANC denial (spearheaded from the top by President Thabo Mbeki) of HIV/AIDS as a major social and medical problem in South Africa. This denial began with the rejection of the Maputo Statement to address the epidemic. It was further evidenced by the breaks in communication between the ANC and leading South African scientists and public health activists who could have been central in making South Africa a leader in fighting HIV/AIDS.[6] It became internationally infamous when Mbeki sought counsel from a group of American scientists known as "AIDS dissidents," who reject the Human Immunodeficiency Virus (HIV) as the cause of HIV/AIDS (Marais, 1999).

But negligence of the needs of poor people with HIV/AIDS was not an isolated anomaly of postapartheid ANC policymaking. Although there is an active debate about exactly why, and to what extent, the ANC government in South Africa so decisively embraced neoliberal economic policies, that they have has been clear since the 1996 Growth, Employment and Redistribution (GEAR) macroeconomic policy plan. This plan focused on controlling inflation, reducing government deficit, controlling spending, and various measures to support exports and attract foreign direct investment. It's main proponents, Mbeki himself and Ministers of finance and Trade played leadership roles in setting economic policy in the new government. As Patrick Bond (2004a) explains, given the fact that negotiated peace in South Africa had left the economic basis of power intact, the ANC government had two options:

> To mobilize the people and all their enthusiasm, energy, and hard work, use a larger share of the economic surplus (through state directed investments and higher taxes), and stop the flow of capital abroad, including the repayment of illegitimate apartheid era debt. The other was to adopt a neoliberal capitalist path, with a small reform here or there, while posturing as if social democracy was on the horizon. (p. 45)

While Mbeki's well-publicized AIDS denialism and public statements that treatments were poison sparked a battle with scientists and AIDS activists, the constraints on public health development imposed by the GEAR policy and the ideology that supported it were an equally important and overlooked barrier to treatment and care for South Africans living with HIV/AIDS.

---

[6]This quote from Prof. Coovadia describes the change in ANC HIV/AIDS approach: "Early on there was no hint of peculiar views. My colleague was the chair of the AIDS directorate, and I was chair of the AIDS advisory committee to government. It became difficult if not impossible to communicate with the minister of health. It was a very good committee too, broadly representative (Everyone you would want. Religious people, pharmacists, blood transfusion). The communication gap was strange because the minister of health had appointed me to head a group to advise on the MTCT issue. And it wasn't an issue of distance, these were colleagues. These were early pin-pricks that came to a head with Sarafina II in 1996. The advisory committee was disbanded under Zuma's reign. They haven't reformed this committee, and now it is a government committee, but you can't have a committee to lead the war against AIDS just by having politicians there" (April, 2002).

Occupational Health of Health Care Workers

What would it mean to address a global public health crisis from a "work environment" perspective? Work-environment policy research begins with a shared understanding of the dynamics of the work environment and the interaction of levels of causation of occupational injury and illness that encompass political, economic, social and historical factors. Levenstein and Wooding assert that the protection of workers depends on a triangle of control between the boss, workers, and any potential hazards, in which the boss holds most of the power over both hazards and the workforce (Wooding & Levenstein, 1999). How this dynamic plays out is affected by the relative power of key social actors and is mediated by race and gender, but class struggle is the bottom line determinant of occupational health and safety.

I was interested in what was particular to health care workers, nurses in the hospital setting. My work as a union organizer in the health care sector in a part of the country undergoing workplace restructuring and reengineering in the mid 1990s had given me a firsthand education in what was driving the current work environment for U.S. nurses and health care workers. Crisis in health care costs had lead to the introduction of managed care, and these contracts had forced hospitals to compete with each other to deliver health care at the lowest cost possible; typically they bid on contracts to deliver "below cost" care (Brannon, 1994). This competition, and the emergence of for-profit players who began to set new industry standards, brought a host of strategies—often implemented by well-known, high-priced consultants—aimed at reducing labor costs. Key to understanding this on the ground was realizing that the language of "improving quality," "patient-focused care," and improved "efficiency" were the lingo of downsizing for the health care industry. This was one effect of the intensified commodification of health care in the United States in the 1990s. The result for nurses was a severe decline in working conditions, which increased occupational health risks, especially due to short-staffing, rotating to unfamiliar jobs, deskilling, cross-training, and the use of temporary employees. In short, all manner of alterations to the work organization of nurses to mitigate the impacts of short-staffed hospitals. I was very interested in how the work organization of nurses defined their working conditions, and how nurses' knowledge of their own jobs held the key to providing the best patient care under the best conditions for work, a kind of marriage between effectiveness, skill, and decent work. And nurses' workplace involvement was expanding due to these industry changes on work organization. Besides an increase in unionizing drives, nurses were involved in many campaigns to improve staffing levels, save public hospitals, and reduce injuries (Brannon,1994). That these campaigns were framed around protecting nurses and improving patient care was a key characteristic of the work environment for health care workers and the range of social actors and forces that could be brought to play.

I thought two characteristics of the U.S. health care work environment for nurses were the most salient for investigation in South Africa. First were the impacts of reforms aimed at increasing productivity and efficiency in the context of increasing commodification of care. In the current era the autonomy of hospitals has been reduced, and their organizations and structures have become highly influenced by changes in the health care industry (Brannon, 1994). The most significant pressures on nurses today originate in the larger health care industry and filter down to nurses through the impact of various reforms on their day-to-day tasks and conditions of work. In sum, the most important outcome is that, for a variety of reasons across contexts, fewer nurses are required to do intensified work.

The second characteristic was the involvement of nurses in fighting these reforms, through unions and other workplace and policy activities, and the generally high level of support and respect that nurses engender. "Social unionism" has been defined as a union movement that fights for social gains, beyond the individual gains for a set of workers in a given workplace (Moody, 1988). In the U.S. context, public-sector employees, notably teachers, have often waged struggles based on their commitment to providing social goods (Johnstone, 1994). In South Africa the preeminence of unions in the fight against apartheid is one of the strongest historical examples of social unionism, and this ethic continues to drive labors rhetoric and strategy in that country (Vavi, 2004). Looking at the dynamics of labor/management relations in South Africa is an important lens through which to examine social unionism in the postapartheid context.

Feminist economists have expanded the idea of the care economy, which is divided into formal and informal sectors (Folbre, Bergmann, Floro, & Agarwal, 1991). The care economy spans informal, unpaid labor in the home to paid formal employment in both public and private sectors. Care is performed primarily by women, and just as low-paid work brings down the price of other labor, the care economy drags down the price paid for formalized work such as nursing by presenting the perpetual option that the work can be externalized to the unpaid, informal sector. Many of the battles within nursing have concerned containing caring tasks within a profession that appear to be the same as those performed by women in the home (Melosch, 1982). Ultimately, how care is produced and reproduced socially is a primary social question that has historically determined much gender-based oppression, and this is a workplace issue as well. For South African nurses, most of them women, this tension between the formal and informal, paid and not, was intensified by the lack of available treatment for HIV/AIDS and the additional burden of caring for the sick, dying, and orphans in the community shouldered by women.

The primary ways of addressing the HIV/AIDS epidemic—prevention, care, treatment, research, policymaking, activism—all assume and require involvement of health care workers. A labor/work-environment approach begins with the recognition of this fact: that the workforce that provides patient care and treatment is the primary component of infrastructure. Attention to the health of patients and communities cannot be separated from the well-being of this workforce and the adequacy of their work environment.

On the other hand, a labor/work-environment approach to public health issues also entails viewing labor as a primary political advocate for the public health system and the population served. This role stems from the intimate relationship between the patient and the caregiver, but is also related to the structural forces that govern this relationship. Health systems that rely on the commitment of caregivers to make up the difference on short-staffed hospital wards, for example, assume that the workforce is sufficiently disempowered to object.

As the story of ARV treatment in developing countries continues to unfold, the values embedded in a labor/work-environment perspective are paramount in the choices about how to address HIV/AIDS. The key issue from a labor/ work-environment approach concerns the ability of people who do the work to have a say in how that work is done and under what conditions. This puts the voices of health care workers up against the range of forces that affect their workplace: the HIV/AIDS epidemic, health sector management, government, and international policymakers and donors.

Conceptual Framework

This book describes the occupational health of South African public-sector hospital nurses in the context of neoliberal globalization and the HIV/AIDS epidemic. This story is important because of the truly pivotal perspective of South African nurses on the HIV/AIDS epidemics, as well as the lessons that it offers about developing effective work-environment policy for health care workers. Chen, Evans, Anand, Brown, Boufford, Chowdhury, et al. (2004) has described the challenges that health workers face in the developing world as a "triple threat"—occupational risk of infection, impacts of HIV/AIDS in their communities and families and their own infections, and the intensification of their jobs due to the epidemic. Henwood and colleagues (2005) advocate for placing nurses' (and other health care workers') occupational health and safety at the center of strengthening nurses and other health workers role in securing workplace rights. They argue that this is the vital missing link in creating a culture of care in health services that is essential to providing care and treatment for people living with HIV/AIDS.

Yet, as Turshen (1999) and Loewenson (1993) describe, health services in Southern Africa have been negatively impacted by structural-adjustment programs and the emphasis on privatization of health services. These developments are not limited to southern Africa; they are part of international trends in both developed and developing countries, which have increased inequality between countries and within them (Navarro, 2004). To understand the challenges that nurses face and their reactions to them, it is necessary to understand the political and economic forces that play a role in determining how health care is delivered, who gains access to quality care, and how workers are treated in the delivery of that care.

This book presents a case study that incorporates many levels of context that are both key parts of the story and part of the framework for analyzing the case. According to Yin, "you would use the case study method because you deliberately wanted to cover contextual conditions" (1994, p. 12). Stake (1995) points out that "qualitative case researchers orient to complexities connecting ordinary practice in natural habitats to the abstractions and concerns of diverse academic disciplines" (p. 38). Overall, this project is best described by Yin's assertion that case studies are most similar to histories of contemporary events.

This study of the occupational health of South African public hospital nurses can be pictured as a "funnel" that moves from large global issues to small local issues. It begins with the aborted efforts of African countries to become healthy, sustainable, independent nations and ends with the health dilemmas facing public-sector hospital nurses in South Africa, who work in underresourced, high HIV-prevalent settings. These local effects are mediated by the political and economic changes that have accompanied neoliberal globalization during the 1980s and 1990s.

The case is presented through a detailed background section that acts as the frame for analysis. This frame is the introduction of neoliberal policies to Africa and South Africa; the impacts on health systems, health workers and health services; and the explosion of the HIV/AIDS epidemic in sub-Saharan Africa. The choice of factors to frame the case study is based on a wide range of literature that identifies the HIV/AIDS epidemic, African history of colonialism and inde-pendence movements, and the influence of neoliberal globalization on health-sector development as the most important factors that determine the hospital work environment (Benatar, 2004; Gish, 2004; Loewenson, 2001; Turshen, 1999).

Diverse case studies have been used to establish the link between neoliberal globalization and a range of bad health effects on communities of poor and working people (Burawoy, Blum, George, Zsuzsa, Thayer, Gowan, et al., 2000; Kim, Millen, Irwin, & Gershman, 2000). These volumes share the premise that documenting the impacts of neoliberal globalization is a key to understanding and changing global forces and balances of power. Burawoy et al. (2000) refers to these case studies as "grounded globalizations," which can be employed to evaluate and understand abstract theories about the effects of neoliberal global-ization, as well as provide clues to building a theory of "globalization from the bottom up." Grounded globalizations are linked by the fact that they document the impact of the set of policies, such as privatization and deregulation that are intended to spur growth and development through the free market.

Another important purpose of the grounded globalization is to give voice to people who are impacted by global forces and usually ignored. One of the characteristics of the global economy is that capital is privileged over workers in its ability to move and control. For example, transnational corporations can far more easily move production to achieve low labor costs than workers can migrate for job opportunities; capital often operates from a position of privileged information and 24-hour surveillance of conditions, while workers are rooted to a particular place and the timing of family life. An important function of the grounded globalization is to assist the workforce in understanding the levels of working conditions that are typically only accessible to capital. Individual and group interviews were used in this project in order to capture the voices of public-sector hospital nurses and managers. These voices were used to "tell the story" of this case in a format that allows the voice to, at least in part, carry the story and connect to the larger issues that are explored.

Chapters 1 and 2 look in-depth at the effects of the globalization of the economy on sub-Saharan Africa in general, and South Africa in particular. These sections describe how economic conditions constrained the possibilities in post-apartheid South Africa and led to inadequate investments in public health driven by neoliberal demands for reductions/constraints in government spending. This, in turn, set the stage for the ravages of HIV/AIDS in southern Africa's economic powerhouse. Chapter 3 looks at the work environment of nurses, and in particular how economic conditions relate to working conditions and increased risk of occupational injury and illness, especially due to staff shortages. Chapters 4 to 6 present a case study of three hospitals in KwaZulu-Natal, South Africa, which examines the occupational health and safety of nurses. In chapter 7 I return to the task of defining a labor/work-environment approach to a global public health issue in light of the situations of particular hospitals charged with meeting the needs of people and communities living with HIV/AIDS in an area experiencing particularly high prevalence of the disease.

CHAPTER 1

∝ ∽

Globalization and Health in sub-Saharan Africa

The story of the occupational health of nurses in KZN, South Africa, needs to be understood in terms of the global forces that impinge on nurses' care for people with HIV/AIDS. The goal of this book is to treat a complex subject in a complex manner. Academic study of and debate about the nature of neoliberal globalization; theories of the work environment; brain drain and the global nursing shortage; the African and South African HIV/AIDS epidemic; and nurses, HIV/AIDS and occupational health are important to developing a rich context. The coverage is not meant to be exhaustive; rather it highlights aspects of the debate that are most salient to this project.

Neoliberal Globalization

Ideology or Legitimate Economic Development Strategy?

Neoliberal globalization, understood as an attempt by an elite group to organize and manage a global free trade/free enterprise economy, makes privatization and monetarism the cornerstones of health policy for developed and developing countries. This is the current context for health-sector development.

Neoliberal globalization refers to the global extension of "free market" principles, and in theory, the integration into one world market (Tabb, 2001). Its proponents have argued that globalization will result in an upward convergence between wages and standards of living between developed and developing countries. Neoliberal policies center on the claim that a free market, through competition and consumer demands, will result in the greatest efficiencies for producing goods and services alike. Basic policy prescriptions aim at reducing regulations on capital and production, privatization, and restraint in state spending (McMichael, 2000). The economic theory supporting neoliberal policy is most associated with Milton Friedman of the University of Chicago (Friedman, 1962), and the driving idea is that the unimpeded market will provide efficiency and maximum profit, and that this course of development will trickle down throughout a society and provide the best distribution of wealth. In the developing world, the International Monetary Fund (IMF), the World Bank, and the World Trade Organization (WTO) have historically been at the forefront of developing and enforcing neoliberal policy packages, notably through Structural Adjustment Programmes and IMF loan conditionalities beginning in the 1980s.

Critics of neoliberal globalization object to policies aimed at expanding the global free market and the claim that the market will be sufficient to solve many social and economic problems. An underlying criticism of neoliberal globalization is that it is an ideology propagated by an elite class masked as economic development theory. This view has been developed critically by an analysis of power in the post-Cold War period, and empirically by pinpointing how evidence used to evaluate the success of neoliberal policies is skewed or ignored.

A relevant example for African postcolonial development is the examination of the case of the so-called Asian Tigers, developed by Arrighi (2002). South Korea's swift economic development is often held up by the World Bank, IMF, WTO, and academic supporters as the model of how neoliberal policies lead to rapid export-based economic growth. The Asian Tiger "model" fails to account for the fact that in actuality, these economies were highly protected through authoritarian, often repressive governments and supported with international preferences. The argument for reduced state involvement and the free market—centerpieces of neoliberal policy—is therefore not supported through this example. Arrighi then offers an alternative explanation that compares development in certain African and Asian countries over specific time periods, which supports his contention that limited opportunities and global conditions were the most important factors in the bifurcation of success in the economic growth of developing countries in different regions of the world.

The Municipal Services Project (MSP) is a research, policy, and education initiative begun in 2000 to examine the restructuring of municipal services in southern Africa. The project's central interests are "the impacts of decentralization, privatization, cost recovery and community participation on the delivery of basic services to the rural and urban poor, and how these reforms impact on public, industrial and mental health" (Municipal Services Project [MSP], 2008). McDonald (2004) describes how the sale of state assets to private firms, and subsequent privatization and partial privatization of water and electricity in South Africa, have not reduced the cost of services, increased their availability, or resulted in economic gains for municipalities, though these outcomes were the explicit claims motivating privatization. Through case studies such as privatization of water services in the Western Cape (South Africa) and Buenos Aires (Argentina), and electricity services in Soweto (Gauteng, South Africa), the MSP builds an empirical base for criticizing the specific tactics of neoliberal policy.

Rowthorn and Kozul-Wright (1998) argue that economic data do not bear the claims of neoliberalism's proponents that domestic policy is irrelevant to development, and that economic growth can hinge on outward-directed policy.

They confirm that domestic policy, including industrial policy, continues to be a key to economic and social development in the developing world, despite the shift in policy trends from "developmentalism" to "globalism" (McMichael, 2000). Mkandawire and Soludo (1999) make the same arguments from the African perspective, noting that state policies and social spending in African counties had made positive impacts before SAPs were introduced. These observations are part of a critical analysis of the harm done when national sovereignty over policymaking is relinquished to global economic interests.

A hallmark of the criticism of neoliberal globalization is that so many people are left out of its benefits and decision-making processes. Navarro (2004) argues that class power and an alliance of elite interests within and between countries is a defining characteristic of this type globalization.

> What now passes as globalization is a specific type of internationalization of capital, labor, and knowledge, characterized by an unrestrained and unregulated search for profits and greatly enhanced by the public policies initiated by the governments of President Reagan and Prime Minister Thatcher and continued by their successors . . . neoliberalism and globalization are the instruments of class domination. (p. 222)

His descriptions of globalization as an ideological projection by a group of self-interested leaders is echoed by McMichael's (2000) description of the "Globalization project" as

> An emerging vision of the world and its resources as a globally organized and managed free trade/free enterprise economy pursued by a largely unaccountable political and economic elite. (p. 354)

Translating this to the postapartheid South African experience, Bond (2000) describes how elites within South Africa's ANC-led government pushed the adoption of neoliberal policies and betrayed the hopes and loyalties of poor and working class South Africans. He analyzes the ANC adoption of neoliberal policies in terms of the formation of a new elite class of black South Africans, formally of the liberation movement, and terms the new terrain in South Africa "class apartheid."

Neoliberal policy trends have also been at the center of debate over health policy. In the 1980s the Reagan government in the United States and the Thatcher government in Britain advocated for commodification and privatization of health care services (Navarro, 2004). This has taken many forms, and no part of the world has been immune to the focus on cost-effectiveness as a key criterion for health systems. Navarro examines how the World Health Organization (WHO), the largest international body devoted to international public health, reproduces the discourse of the market in health care based on the private U.S. model, despite evidence to the contrary that shows how market-based health policies have resulted in millions of uninsured in the United States, and the dissatisfaction of the vast majority of people with their health care. The WHO, along with the World Bank and IMF, has played a key role in exporting these policies to the developing world beginning in the 1980s (Turshen, 1999). Turshen carefully documents the impacts of privatization policies on health services in Africa, concluding that they have resulted in an overall disinvestment in health.

The HIV/AIDS epidemic exploded in southern Africa during the period of globalization, structural adjustment programs, and neoliberal reforms. Just a few decades prior, many African countries newly independent from colonial rule, held out the promise of better life and health. Indeed, during the late 1950s and the 1960s great improvements were made in such things as life expectancy and infant mortality. In the 1970s state-led national development was replaced by the push for participation in the global economy (McMichael, 2000). Beginning in the 1980s (SAPs), brought about by neoliberal globalization, destroyed the capacity of African countries to determine their own social spending, and thus to build working health systems (Gloyd, 2004; Mkandawire & Soludo, 1999; Turshen 1999). The adoption of neoliberal economic and social policies had grave consequences for public health and health services in southern African countries and is one key to understanding the explosion of the HIV/AIDS epidemic in sub-Saharan Africa. The withering of the public health infrastructure had profound consequences for frontline health care workers, especially nurses.

Neoliberalism[1] came to Africa via the World Bank (WB) and International Monetary Fund (IMF). Structural Adjustment Programs introduced in the 1980s in the context of the African "Debt Crisis" demanded policy reforms that, although aimed primarily at economic growth, affected all areas of development (Mkandawire & Soludo, 1999). Because within the orthodoxy of neoliberalism the free market provides the most efficient and productive way to fund and deliver social goods, economic growth was given a central position in all policy areas, including health and education. Since the neoliberal view sees much of the public sector as a distortion of the free market, this set of policies amounted to a specific attack on publicly financed and supplied social goods like education and health care.

Health and Development in sub-Saharan Africa

Many of the SSA countries achieved independence from colonial rule in the 1960s and 1970s. The ideals of liberal democracy and human rights, refashioned by Africans from the traditions of colonizers and then used against them during

---

[1] Defined in the previous chapter, and illustrated by this quote from McMichael (2000): An emerging vision of the world and its resources as a globally organized and managed free trade/free enterprise economy pursued by a largely unaccountable political and economic elite (p. 354).

independence struggles, placed the language of rights and equality at the center of independence struggles (McMichael, 2000). The international black power movement and the socialist example fed the formation of fledgling nation states. Despite ethnic differences and borders drawn by colonists, independence movements were intensely nationalistic. Bond (2001) comments on how nationalist movements used democratic principles as their rallying points:

> The language of the nationalist movement was the language of democracy, as is clear from: I Speak of Freedom (Nyerere), Without Bitterness (Orizu), Facing Mount Kenya (Kenyatta), Not Yet Uhuru (Odinga), Freedom and Development (Nyerere), African Socialism (Senghor), and The Wretched of the Earth (Fanon). It denounced the violation of dignity of the colonized, the denial of basic rights, the political disenfranchisement of the colonized, racial discrimination, lack of equal opportunity and equal access, and economic exploitation of the colonized. The people were mobilized according to these grievances and expectations of a more democratic dispensation. (p. 45)

Independence meant that SSA states could begin to define their own development trajectory. Import Substitution Industrialization[2] (ISI) was adopted in sub-Saharan African countries to compensate for the colonial division of labor, which had relegated them to producers of primary commodity exports (Mkandawire & Soludo, 1999). This policy direction was predicated on terms of trade decline for primary commodity exporters. ISI was supported by policies such as exchange-rate manipulation, import tariffs, and subsidization of industry that were intended to protect fledgling industries. ISI was the "economic orthodoxy" in the postwar Latin America (McMichael, 2000), and it was widely followed in independent African states.

At least a portion of the revenues derived from import-substitution manufacturing was invested in the nation. Even with high levels of corruption, most nations began a vigorous program of social spending on such things as health care and education (Schoepf, Schoepf, & Millen, 2000). In addition, states were encouraged by the IMF and the WB to borrow billions for major infrastructure programs like dams, hydroelectric power plants, highways, and airports (Bond, 2001).

SSA countries made substantial gains in this period. In some countries primary school enrollment increased by as much as 25%. The industrialization process, however incomplete, added infrastructure and developed workforce skills in management and administration (Mkandawire & Soludo, 1999). Health systems were expanded (Turshen, 1999). The improved HDI ranking of SSA countries in this period reflects these improvements (Arrighi, 2002).

---

[2]National industrial development policy that allows nations to produce what they formerly had to import.

The approach that African countries took to development was a mirror of the approach to development in first- and second-world countries across differences in political systems. Industrialization was a key policy area for securing economic independence and political legitimacy (McMichael, 2000). Political legitimacy came as a result of meeting social needs for education, health, and basic services.

Development efforts had transnational and international aspects. African countries made strides to band together with other developing countries to change the parameters of world economic order, examine the social needs of citizens, and address terms of trade imbalances (Arrighi, 2002). In 1967 the group of 77 (G77) was formed in an effort to create one voice for third world nations at the United Nations Conference for Trade and Development (UNCTAD) in Algiers (Tabb, 2001). The New International Economic Order (NIEO) was developed as an instrument to, in the words of the late Tanzanian president Julius K. Nyerere, "complete the liberation of third world countries from external domination" (Nyerere, 1979). The Organization of African Unity (OAU) was formed in 1963 to support liberation struggles in Africa. By the 1970s its mission had come to include mutual support for postindependence development goals based on unity and solidarity within the region (Arrighi, 2002).

Health System Development

Health system development in the independence era occurred atop the history of colonialism (Gish, 2004). Colonization and the slave trade brought diseases and social disruption to Africa. As the colonies produced food that replaced food production of working-class Europeans turned industrial laborers, the amount of food produced for local consumption fell, causing hunger and malnourishment. The Western medical approach to health was imported by colonists, but was not widely available for ailing Africans. At the same time, traditional systems, practitioners, and indigenous understanding of health were interrupted. Over time, systems emerged that embodied the dictates and ideology of colonialism. This meant first-rate Western medicine for whites, public health measures to stop the spread of disease to whites (but not to promote the health of Africans), and care for black laborers insofar as it supported economic interests (Gish, 2004).

Colonial health systems were centered on the urban hospital, located where the largest nonnative populations lived (Turshen, 1999). The government hospital was also essential to colonial rule and often operated as an extension of the military. Rural dispensaries, typically run by missionaries, offered drugs and basic maternity services. Investment in the health of native populations was marginal (Banerji, 2004; Gish, 2004). After independence, many African governments extended these inherited health services, and did not change the basic focus of the Western model (Schoepf et al., 2000). This meant that weaknesses in addressing public health, limited rural access, and lack of community input were often reproduced (Gish, 2004):

Often leaders of newly independent countries, and, more particularly, the medical leadership, did not question the essential character of the health services they had inherited. Instead, they aspired to spread these services to the whole of the population. The new services were to be "high standard," as defined by the medical elite, and at the same time serve the needs of the whole population. More often than not though, it was the prestigious hospital plan that was approved and built, and not the health centers, rural clinics, or preventative programs. The post-independence period, then, often saw a continuation of more of the same kind of health system that operated under colonial rule—a system in which the rural poor was provided limited care and services only after the needs of the urban elite was attended to. (p. 23)

However, the concept of "colonial legacy" is complex. Health care infra-structure was also a positive feature of the colonial legacy. In some African countries, such as Zimbabwe, a public health system modeled on the British National Health Service provided the skeleton of a system that could be universalized (Turshen, 1999). Many countries set out to provide access to public health care; in so doing, they followed the public model of the colonial powers, not the private U.S. system.

In 1978 there was a watershed event in international public health policy. The Alma-Ata Conference (named for its location in Kazakhstan) was organized by the World Health Organization (WHO) and UNICEF, and coalesced around a community--based, public health approach dubbed primary health care (PHC) (WHO, 1978). One of the most radical aspects of PHC was that it was designed to apply to developing and industrialized countries alike. This was not "primitive" health care for the resource-poor, but a universal program based on sound public health principles.

The WHO commitment to PHC grew out of their experiences with the failure of developing countries to adapt vertical programs—so named because of their bureaucratic organization and single purpose—to rural conditions and third world economies (Banerji, 1984). The WHO had advised countries to build up basic health services at the clinic level as a means to consolidate the gains in health improvements brought by vertical programs to alleviate TB and malaria (among other diseases). However, these attempts failed in part because competition between vertical services and clinics led to staff and resource shortages, and training and management problems. The management and skills needed for a vertical program that focuses on a single disease, and often a single intervention such as immunization or a short course of treatment, is different from what is required to maintain community health over time. PHC entailed a horizontally integrated system that addressed contextual issues and involved community.

The PHC approach was based on the innovations made in former colonies and other situations where health outcomes were strongly linked to economic exploitation and inequality (Hong, 2004). For example, The Barefoot Doctor program in China integrated community-led health and traditional medicine (Hong, 2004), and postindependence Tanzania developed equity-based programs that emphasized the socioeconomic determinants of disease (Turshen, 1999). In South Africa, community-oriented primary care (COPC) was pioneered by Emily and Sidney Kark at a clinic in Pholela (Kark & Cassel, 2002; Kark & Kark, 1983; Susser, 1999). Kark's work at Pholela addressed the role that the apartheid labor system played in contributing to the spread of sexually transmitted disease (a direct foreshadowing of the context of migrant labor for the spread of HIV/AIDS). H. Jack Geiger went to Pholela as a medical student to work with Kark, and brought the COPC model to the American South, where race/class "apartheid" (and the resulting labor conditions) also determined health (Geiger, 2002). While Kark's work had little influence on the apartheid-era health system overall, it became the basis for an indigenous progressive public health movement in South Africa that made huge contributions to postapartheid health policy (Susser, 1999).

The Alma-Ata declaration defines health as a "state of complete physical, mental, and social wellbeing" and a human right for which governments are responsible (WHO, 1978). It posits that inequality is an unacceptable condition for health and begins with the premise that poor health is a direct result of poverty. It refers specifically to the New International Economic Order (NIEO), proposed by the G77 in the 1970s, as a tool for reducing inequality. The declaration explicitly states the right and duty of people to participate in the planning and implementation of health care. The declaration laid out a framework for PHC that required national governments to develop a plan for health, and the goal of an acceptable level of health for all people by the year 2000. Most important, the resolutions at Alma-Ata recognized that the politics of health were inseparable from the technical questions of how health care, services, and prevention were developed and provided.

Technically, PHC is based on a referral system from primary to secondary levels of health care, and above as needed (Hong, 2004; Turshen, 1999). This decentralized system aims to assure the availability of services at the local level while reducing expenditures in high-level, typically urban-based, hospitals. It involves intense community participation at the local level, and incorporates traditional and preventative health services. The system is dependent on horizontal integration of a variety of levels and types of services, as opposed to single-focused, separately managed vertical programming. Horizontal integration is the province of government because of its power to oversee planning across diverse sites and institutions.

Some independent African countries had what Turshen term "remarkable success" (1999, p. 25) implementing PHC. Zimbabwe gained independence in 1980 and quickly moved to increase access to health care for rural populations and the percentage of the health budget allocated to preventive care. The number of rural health centers doubled, and immunizations and clinic births increased.[3] Life

---

[3] One factor in the decline in infant mortality and childbirth-related death in mothers.

expectancy in Zimbabwe increased (from 55 to 60 years), child malnutrition fell (from 22% to 12%), and infant mortality dropped from 100 to 53 per 1000 live births (Turshen, 1999).

Countries with fewer resources than Zimbabwe also managed some success with PHC. Zambia's constitution after independence in 1964 forbade charging for health care, and one of government's first efforts was to extend health services. Between 1965 and 1981 the ratios of doctors and nurses to population were reduced by 50% to 70%, though urban bias remained. The government's investment in health increased, and in 1979 PHC was formally adopted (Loewenson, 1993). Mozambique was poor at independence in 1975; few health facilities existed, and most doctors had immigrated to Portugal. Remarkably, even in these conditions and in the context of a guerilla war, the government ran successful mass campaigns for immunization and environmental sanitation, and extended free care through PHC. The numbers of PHC clinics and health care workers improved significantly, and care was extended to rural populations (Turshen, 1999).

Debt Crisis

In the beginning of the 1970s the world economy and the global balance of power created conditions that were favorable for African development (Bond, 2000; Habib & Padeyachee, 2000; Tabb, 2001). Increased productivity and trade in the post–World War II era increased international competition and decreased the power of the United States. The social and economic costs of the failure to win the war in Vietnam contributed to deterioration of U.S. hegemony and raised hopes that the third world could stand up to the world's superpowers (Arrighi, 2002). The formation of OPEC reinforced this hope. Economic conditions favored developing countries, and terms of trade improved. Excess liquidity based on petrodollars was recycled as loan capital, which was made available to second- and third-world countries at highly favorable rates. Loans were actively and aggressively marketed to developing countries and were taken to fund the post-colonial expansion (McMichael, 2000).

By the end of the 1970s the conditions that had been favorable for Africa's postindependence expansion changed (Arrighi, 2002). The oil crises that marked the end of the decade had disastrous results for Africa as commodity prices collapsed. The United States adopted strict monetarist policies and shifted from the largest creditor to the largest debtor nation, and African countries came into competition with the economic giant (as well as all other developing regions) for increasingly scarce investment. African borrowers were left with serious balance-of-payment difficulties. The aggressive decision by the IMF and WB to help global banks recover the loans they made to developing countries in the 1970s and early 1980s prompted the debt crisis (Arrighi, 2002; McMichael, 2000; Mkandawire & Soludo, 1999).

The Bretton Woods Institutions played the role of collection agency for global capital. Countries could not pay, got behind, and then were forced by the IMF to accept conditionalities that required them to give up their hard-won sovereignty over social and economic policy if they were to receive loans (McMichael, 2000; Mkandawire & Soludo, 1999). This marked the end of a brief period of national development, and the beginning of a period of policymaking controlled by the IMF and World Bank.

African Policy Response to the Debt Crisis

African leaders attempted to respond to the debt crisis on their own terms. In 1980 African leaders met in Nigeria under the OAU and drafted the Lagos Plan of Action for the Economic Development of Africa, 1980–2000 (Organization of African Unity [OAU], 1980). The Lagos Plan blamed the crisis on deteriorating terms of trade, protectionism of wealthy countries, interest rates, and debt-servicing obligations. The plan proposed at Lagos saw the resolution of the crisis on increasing self-reliance and integration of national resources. In short, Lagos was critical of the world-market mechanisms for their role in the crisis, and sought relief from harsh external conditions.

At the same time that OAU leaders met in Lagos, the World Bank published a report that spelled out their assessment of the causes of the debt crisis and the steps African countries needed to take to address them (Berg, 1981). Known as the Berg report, for its main author, this document attributed the debt crisis to national industrial development policies. The report made recommendations that became the basis of the structural adjustment programs that were offered in generic form to developing countries. Recommendations included privatization of both industry and social services. Another influential paper at the time vilified the role of corrupt leaders in using industrialization and economic control inherited from colonial regimes for their own personal benefit (Bates, 1981). This view justified the marginalization of African leadership in solving the debt crisis.

In 1984 the OAU and the UN produced a joint document on economic recovery that capitulated to the "internalist" analysis—analysis that placed the blame for the debt crisis on the African states' leadership and policies rather than external forces—by acknowledging African governments' responsibility for the crisis, and more pointedly, the need for international assistance (UNDESA, 1986). In a departure from the Lagos plan, it agreed to implement many recommendations of the Berg report and asked in exchange that the international community assist in easing debt burden and raise the price paid for exports. This last ditch attempt at proactive policymaking by the OAU failed.

The bailout that followed benefited private lenders in danger of losing their investments, not struggling Africans. Between 1984 and 1996 the lowest income African countries repaid $1.5 billion, a sum 1.5 times that owed in 1980. Repayment averaged 16% of African government spending during the 1980s, compared with 1% on education, 10% on defense, and 4% on health (Mkandawire & Soludo, 1999).

Despite the fact that African countries had followed an accepted strategy for development—industrialization and investment in social goods—these measures were blamed for the debt crisis to the exclusion of external factors. A new mode of development and neoliberal globalization was introduced through the SAPs (McMichael, 2000). This had serious impacts on health and health services.

At the same time that industrial policy came under attack in Africa, the PHC movement also met powerful resistance. The ultraconservative Heritage Foundation quickly attacked the Alma-Ata declaration, particularly the allegiance to the NIEO stated in the declaration (Turshen, 1999). In the early 1980s USAID and the World Bank began to advance a competing strategy that was a better ideological fit with the Berg report and SAPs called "selective strategies" (Banerji, 1984). Selective strategies was based on the view that most health care is best delivered and financed privately, and that the public sector should engage in only selective areas of last resort. A battle ensued on the theoretical and programmatic side between PHC and selective strategies, based principally upon the issue of scarcity of resources and cost-effectiveness (Turshen, 1999).

By the 1980s the mounting debt crisis, the power of the SAPs, and World Bank guidelines for health policy interrupted the progress of PHC. The "dreams of equality" expressed at Alma-Ata (Turshen, 1999, p. 3) were deferred as countries were forced to grapple with the imperative for economic efficiency." In 1982 UNICEF split from the WHO and joined the World Bank and USAID in introducing selective strategies as an affordable alternative to comprehensive PHC (Banerji, 1999). Aid-package conditionalities came to include clauses that governed health care financing (Turshen, 1999):

> Borrowing the idiom of equity and efficiency, the promoters of selective strategies used the budgetary crisis to virtually force acceptance of alternative financing schemes for health services as part of larger packages of economic reform, upon which all aid was made contingent. At the macro-economic level, the new health plans were part of much wider proposals to privatize all sectors of the economy. (p. 44)

Impacts of the SAPs on Health

Zimbabwean public health researcher and activist Rene Loewenson (1993) recounts a conversation between two workers concerning the Zimbabwean economic structural adjustment program (ESAP):

> My Friend, I've been working all week and now I'm going home with money that will not even buy food for a day. This ESAP is a bitter pill. It's like swallowing ten chloroquin tablets without water.
> It's Extreme Suffering of African People
> I was retrenched last month, and now I can't find a job anywhere
> It's not suffering for all African people, look at that Mercedes going by.
> It's extreme state applied poverty. (p. 718)

According to the World Bank, Structural Adjustment Programs (SAPs) were designed to "unleash markets so that competition can help improve the allocation of resources . . . getting price signals right and creating a climate that allows businesses to respond to those signals in ways that increase return on investments" (World Bank, 1993, p. 7). The economic policies of the SAP reflected the neoliberal orthodoxy that liberating the free market would be sufficient to solve both economic and social problems. As Loewenson observes (1993),

> The SAPs were austerity measures, in line with the Washington Consensus, designed to liberate public funds for debt repayment and to improve the conditions for local businesses to export goods to gain foreign currency. According to the IMF, SAPs would jump start the economic engines of the poor countries so they would be able to generate sufficient resources to raise standards of living. (p. 721)

Standards of living fell and in practice, the poor, especially women and children, bore the brunt of World Bank imposed austerity (Millen & Holtz, 2000). Cuts in services created greater family need and increased women's burdens as they struggled to care for themselves and their children. In SSA per capita incomes fell by 25% during the 1980s, and unemployment increased (Mkandawire & Soludo, 1999). Not surprisingly, during the 1980s, as more capital flowed out of Africa than in, the gap between rich and poor widened (McMichael, 2000).

The impact of the SAP/World Bank approach on health and health services in Africa can be broadly captured by two terms: disinvestment and privatization. The World Bank approach to health services is spelled out in two policy documents: the 1987 health services financing (World Bank, 1987) and the 1993 World Development Report: Investing in Health (World Bank, 1993). The SAPs had required reductions in social spending that were justified under the economic theory of fiscal responsibility, reducing government deficit, and freeing funds for debt repayment. Underlying this was the belief in the efficiency of the private sector and the rationalizing effects of the market. The World Bank reports of 1987 and 1993 apply these arguments specifically to the health sector and provide a variety of options for privatization and cost recovery in health services. They incorporate the language of selective strategies for the health needs of the poor, as described below (World Bank, 1993):

> Ensuring basic public health services and essential clinical care while the rest of the health system becomes self-financing will require substantial health systems reforms and reallocations of public spending. Only by reducing or eliminating spending on discretionary clinical services can government concentrate on ensuring cost-effective clinical care for the poor. (p. 11)

The disinvestment in government health services is the direct result of the reductions in all social spending and deep cuts to the civil-service workforce required by the SAPs. Access to health care was limited and even when it was available, quality suffered (Turshen, 1999). The retrenchment of health care workers resulted in work intensification and staff shortages. Cuts in wages and labor deregulation meant that remaining workers often toiled under deteriorating conditions. Turshen (1999) also notes that disinvestment in public services is in itself a privatization strategy: "The decline of state services virtually ensures privatization, as ill-paid health personnel pressure the government to liberalize private practice" (Turshen, 1999, p. 45).

Privatization's Impact on Health Care Delivery

The primary impact of privatization on care delivery is the reduction of funding and provision of public health care programs, and methods aimed to increase efficiency and the ability of programs to recoup costs.

When methods to capture costs such as user fees are introduced, the projected intake of funds is often considered "budgeted" money (Arhin-Tenkorang, 2000). In reality, user fees have universally reduced demand, and have failed to collect anything near the proportion they were predicted to (Turshen, 1999).

Redirecting of all social spending and social administration of programs toward financial reforms is another form of disinvestment. The focus on macro-economic policy at the expense of all other areas of planning means that managerial expertise is not directed toward health planning (Mkandawire & Soludo, 1999). Cost-efficiency measures replace health system management.

In the neoliberal view, privatization achieves quality, efficiency, and the proper allocation of resources. The main forms of privatization implemented in the African health sector are user charges, self-financing insurance, private-sector investment, and decentralization (Loewenson, 1993; Turshen, 1999). User fees were intended to capture payment from those who could afford it, and redistribute these funds to pay for health care for the poor. Promoting insurance was meant to increase the ability of Africans to pay for health care, as public care increased in cost to equal private care. Private-sector investment transfers public funds to the private sector and increases competitiveness while allowing the private sector to do the work. Decentralization entails allowing the components of state health systems to act as individual units and apply market incentives to motivate staff and allocate resources, a counter to centralized planning, budget, and administration.

However, the empirical grounds to privatize health care in Africa do not appear to justify such a move. User fees have been shown to reduce use and have failed to yield returns that are reinvested in health financing (Loewenson, 1993). Insurance is out of reach to the poor and, where it exists as a viable market, often serves to reinforce divisions and promote two-tiered systems of care (People's Budget Campaign, 2004). Private practice reinforces the two-tiered systems and promotes a curative-care system with all the implications that this brings (McCoy, Chopra, Loewenson, Aitken, Ngulube, Muula, et al., 2005). Quality and cost are unregulated and unevaluated, and the government investment made through education of practitioners is forfeited in the private sector.

Privatization impacts health services through effects on general public health. Reductions in government spending and privatization of health and other social goods, including basic services like water and electricity, have reduced access to these goods, which has contributed to sickness and disease (Millen & Holtz, 2000). Reductions in food security increased health care demand by increasing illness (Watkinson & Makgetla, 2002). Increases in demand compound the effects of declining access.

Has privatization accomplished what its proponents intended? There can be little argument that the increased poverty in Africa over the last 25 years is associated with specific declines in health indicators. In other words, SAPs have failed to build on the progress made in many African countries during the 1960s and early 1970s. Infant mortality has risen, and life expectancy has fallen (Turshen, 1999). Diseases such as TB and HIV/AIDS have reached epidemic proportions; HIV/AIDS (a relatively new development) and TB (a disease with long history) though in decline in some areas and now strongly resurgent as an OI of HIV infection. Diseases that were thought to be eradicated or rare have reemerged (Loewenson, 1993). And process indicators, such as health service utilization, have shown a decrease associated with fees and reduced availability of services and resources (Turshen, 1999).

If poverty is considered as a cause of poor health and therefore a health indicator, then the health outlook for SSA is especially dire. By the year 2000, 40% of the world's poor resided in sub-Saharan Africa, where only 10% of the world's population lives (United Nations Development Programme [UNDP], 2004).

South Africa and sub-Saharan Africa

While high levels of industrialization and technology cause South Africa to stand out among its neighbors, many indicators show how South Africa fits within the regional context (UNDP, 2004). Disaggregating South African data between rural and urban/industrial centers eliminates most distinctions in indicators between South Africa and neighboring countries: the rural poor in South Africa are as poor as their neighbors in nearby southern African countries, though the in-country inequality is greater (UNDP, 2003).

The United Nations Development Program introduced the Human Development Indicators (HDI)[4] as a counterbalance to the preeminence of economic indicators in measuring development (Fort, Mercer, & Gish, 2004). The HDI index provides a clear means of comparing so-called growth indicators with social

---

[4]The HDI is a composite index for comparing how successful a nation or group is in meeting its human needs. The three main variables embodied in the HDI are life expectancy, literacy, and purchasing power. The HDI of a country varies between zero and one, the closer to one the closer a country is to meeting human needs.

and poverty indicators within the same countries and has provided some famous incongruities. For example, while the United States has the strongest economy, it ranks below Cuba on infant mortality (UNDP, 2004). The HDIs incorporate data from a variety of sources and are comparable over time, despite the fact that some indicators are based on estimates and reflect lack of data or poor data collection.[5]

It is useful to contrast South African, SSA, and developing-country indicators. South Africa exceeds SSA and the developing world on infant and under-5 mortality rates. GDP figures are nearly six times those of SSA, and three times those of other developing countries. Education rates are over 20% better than SSA, and 13% better than the developing-country average. The use of the Internet and cell phones dwarfs the use of modern communications in the rest of SSA. However, at 0.684, the aggregate HDI index figure ranks South Africa 111 and barely exceeds the developing-country aggregate. Despite better infant/under-5 mortality rates, life expectancy in South Africa is very near to the rest of SSA, and dropping. Probability of living until age 65 is low for both males and females, especially low for females considering the normally longer life expectancy. Rates of HIV and TB, the most common opportunistic infection in South Africa, are extremely high. HIV prevalence, at over 20% nationally, exceeds the prevalence in SSA, as do TB cases. Based on the information utilized for the HDI index, the HIV/AIDS epidemic appears to largely explain South Africa's poor rating.

South Africa's index trend (see Table 1) shows that it has returned to a human-development rating at 1980 levels. Since 1995 upward-development trends have reversed directions. This contrasts to other developing countries that have made progress over this same time period.

A look at key Millennium Development Goal progress indicators (see Table 2) shows that reducing South Africa's HDI decline solely to the HIV/AIDS epidemic is misleading. For example, though certainly higher than some places, South

Table 1. Human Development Index Trends 1975-2001

Country	1975	1980	1985	1990	1995	2001
South Africa	0.660	0.676	0.702	0.734	0.741	0.684
China	0.521	0.554	0.591	0.624	0.679	0.721
Indonesia	0.464	0.526	0.528	0.619	0.650	0.682

Source: United Nations Development Programme [UNDP], 2004.

[5]For instance, HIV prevalence estimates have been updated this year with figures that reflect refinement of estimate techniques. Many indicators provide a range to reflect uncertainties.

Table 2. South Africa's Progress toward Millennium Goals

	1990		2000	
MDG, Target and indicator	Rural %	Urban %	Rural %	Urban %
Goal 7, Target 10: Population with improved access to safe drinking water	73	99	73	99
Goal 7, Target 11: Urban population with access to improved sanitation	93		93	

Source: United Nations Development Programme [UNDP], 2003.

Africa has failed to make progress on population access to safe water and improved sanitation. Lack of progress is striking given that in this time period the government changed from one that was racially segregated and based on unequal service provisions, to one that promised improved living standards to Africans. Water privatization has reduced access to safe water in some places, and the use of bucket-system toilets is still prevalent in the townships.

CHAPTER 2

CR SO

Neoliberalism in Postapartheid South Africa and the HIV/AIDS Epidemic

South Africa achieved independence/democracy a couple of decades after many other countries in the region. Independence occurred in the context of global recession, the collapse of the state socialism, and the introduction of structural adjustment programs elsewhere on the continent (Habib & Padayachee, 2000). Highly industrialized and rich in state assets, at independence the new government had economic advantages relative to other SSA countries at the time of their independence (Bond, 2000). Redistribution of these economic advantages to its people had always been a central goal of South Africa's antiapartheid movement. This goal is expressed in the 1955 Freedom Charter, a guiding document for the African National Congress (ANC, 1955):

> The national wealth of our country, the heritage of South Africans, shall be restored to the people;
>
> The mineral wealth beneath the soil, the Banks and monopoly industry shall be transferred to the ownership of the people as a whole;
>
> All other industry and trade shall be controlled to assist the wellbeing of the people;
>
> All people shall have equal rights to trade where they choose, to manufacture and to enter all trades, crafts and professions.

However, the negotiated peace settlement between the apartheid government and the ANC established a very high level of continuity between the old and new South Africa, and redistribution policies were slow in coming (Bond, 2004a). For example, universal health insurance became free care for mothers and children under 6, and land redistribution, a bureaucratic process that has yet to satisfy, forcibly removed communities. Enmeshed in the World Bank consensus, ANC leaders who had come from Congress of South African Trade Unions (COSATU), the United Democratic Front (UDF), and the South African Communist Party (SACP) soon became the proponents of neoliberal economic policies (Bond, 2000).

In 1994, around the same time that the ANC came to power with a landslide victory in the country's first democratic elections, the first cases of heterosexually spread HIV/AIDS were identified in South Africa, foretelling the HIV/AIDS epidemic that would swiftly become a devastating social problem for the country. The HIV/AIDS epidemic exploded in South Africa in the postapartheid period. In 1994 HIV prevalence was estimated at 1%. In the decade that followed, prevalence estimates reached as high as 37% in some areas, with far higher concentrations in particular communities (UNAIDS, 2004). While it is clear that the current government of South Africa inherited the HIV/AIDS epidemic to a large degree, policies since 1994 have exacerbated the conditions for the epidemic and its spread. Economic policies have failed to address poverty, inequality, lack of access to basic services and health care. The lack of antiretroviral treatment (ART) for the poor has led to increased mortality and further spread of AIDS (Abdool-Karim & Abdool-Karim, 2002; Willan, 2004).

After independence, South Africa's rich history of progressive public health contributed to the swift development of health policy aimed at redressing the inequalities of the apartheid era and adoption of a model of district based-primary health care (Stack & Hlela, 2002). However, neoliberal policy and the HIV/AIDS epidemic created harsh conditions for implementing these policies. Because of cuts in public health spending, the public health system was forced to provide care to growing numbers of the poor.

The Apartheid Legacy

One aspect of the legacy of Apartheid is the lack of basic infrastructure for the majority of Africans, especially those living in rural areas, former homelands. The apartheid system was set up to achieve maximum exploitation of labor with minimum social costs. Africans were relegated to townships, homelands, or hostels. Minimal or no services such as water, electricity, education, housing, or health care were provided (Marais, 1999). The most powerful industry, mining, relied on a system of migrant labor where men lived in hostels, returning home periodically to wives and children. This caused social disruption and, as Kark (1950) noted in relation to the syphilis epidemic of the 1930s–1940s, facilitated the spread of communicable disease (Kark & Cassel, 2002).

The history of the struggle against apartheid spans decades and culminates in negotiations and a "peaceful"[1] transition to democracy in the early 1990s.

---

[1] There was no violent overthrow of the government, and negotiations were peaceful. However, violence was extensive in particular areas, especially KZN.

Economic policy was central to these negotiations for the following reasons: development needs for the poor African majority in the new South Africa were urgent; placating capitalists so that they did not withdraw their finances was a priority; and the global economy, economic crisis of the 1980s, and recent recession made economic worries a priority (Adelzadeh, 1996; Bond, 2002; Habib & Padayachee, 2000).

In the 1960s South Africa's growth rate on average was among the highest in the world, along with Japan, Brazil, and South Korea (Arrighi, 2002). The economy under apartheid achieved many of the goals of "import substitution" through state policies that protected industry and particular segments of the workforce (Habib & Padayachee, 2000). By the early 1970s growth trends slowed as the economy faced crisis due to overaccumulation and the impacts of external shocks. In the 1980s the government and business turned to the same strategies for competitiveness undertaken internationally. There were serious splits among Afrikaner capitalists between the "enlightened," who saw the need to expand internationally to solve problems of small markets at home and who wanted to join the global economic system, and the traditionalists who wanted to continue to use state power and resources to protect the economy and white constituents (Bond, 2000).

At the time of transition from apartheid rule to democracy, the world was marked by economic crisis and the end of state socialism. These factors constrained the outcomes of negotiations during government transition. From March 1989 until May 1993 South Africa experienced a severe recession that resulted in dramatic job loss in the formal sector and a huge increase in informal work. By the early 1990s between 40% and 45% of the economically active population found work outside of the formal sector (Adelzadeh, 1996).

In the late 1980s the collapse of the Soviet Union and the destruction of the Berlin wall marked the end of the Cold War period. This resulted in the disappearance of the Soviet bloc funding stream, alliance and support that had supported African independence in general, and the ANC in exile in particular (Bond, 2000). As Trevor Manuel, former leader of the United Democratic Front and soon to be Minister of Finance put it (Marais, 1999),

> The collapse of the Soviet Union, the destruction of the Berlin Wall broke the . . . revolutionary illusions of many. That very stark collapse shifted the debate very significantly. (p. 89)

As economic negotiations played out, neoliberal economic positions began to be favored by the ANC. The ANC ignored a social democratic economic policy package commissioned and released in 1993 (van Ameringen, 1995). The competing model introduced by the "enlightened" faction of the apartheid government in 1993 featured the concept of "growth with redistribution" (Habib & Padayachee, 2000). Although this policy package was roundly attacked for benefiting the white minority, it is similar to the economic policy that the ANC introduced in 1996. As negotiations over economic policy played out, key economic decisions were made without the substantive participation of key leaders, such as those from the Congress of South African Trade Unions (COSATU) and the South African Communist Party (SACP)[2] (Bond, 2000).

Bond (2000, 2004a) points to events that foretold the direction of the new ANC government. The first act of the interim government—the government formed of the ANC and National Party in the months before the 1994 election—was to accept an $850 million IMF loan. Conditonalities for this loan were the same as those imposed on other countries in the region: lower import tariffs, cuts in state spending, and large cuts in public-sector wages. Prior to this, South Africa was free of the conditionalities that burdened their neighbors. In addition to the IMF loan, Bond points to three other decisions that contributed to the shift to neoliberalism. These were the decision to drop the term "nationalization" from ANC rhetoric (1992); to repay $25 billion inherited apartheid-era foreign debt; and to grant the central bank formal independence (1993) (Bond, 2004, pp. 45-46).

Although transition occurred with constraints, the ANC government had legitimate policy options in 1993. As Bond (2004) describes it:

> There were only two basic paths that the ANC could follow. One was to mobilize the people and all their enthusiasm, energy and hard work, use a larger share of the economic surplus (through state-directed investments and higher taxes), and stop the flow of capital abroad, including the repayment of illegitimate apartheid era debt. The other was to adopt a neoliberal capitalist path, with a small reform here or there, while posturing as if social democracy was on the horizon. (p. 45)

From the RDP to GEAR

The ANC-led government pursued a policy package that some have termed "home-grown structural adjustment" (Bond, 2004a; Saul, 2001). This package includes trade liberalization, removal of tariffs, incentives such as free enterprise zones for private capital, removing restrictions on capital mobility, privatization of public assets, and abandoning cross-subsidization (a system where wealthy users subsidize poorer users) in favor of cost-recovery (user fees) for such basics as water and electricity (Habib & Padayachee, 2000). These policies were solidified in the 1996 Growth, Employment and Redistribution macroeconomic policy (GEAR) (Republic of South Africa [RSA], 1996).

GEAR ostensibly replaced the 1994 Reconstruction and Development Programme (RDP) (Bond, 2000). The RDP was drafted through a democratic process in the early days of the birth of the new South African democracy and

---

[2]The SACP, COSATU, and ANC are part of a tripartite alliance, forged in the liberation era, that now operates as a coalition that supports the ANC political party.

became the platform for the ANC in the first election in 1994. Though a close read of the RDP reveals inconsistencies, particularly between fiscal and social policy, this essentially social democratic document became symbolic of participatory democracy and transformation in the new South Africa (ANC, 1992). Marais (1999) describes how GEAR supplanted the RDP:

> The GEAR strategy remains the centre-piece of South Africa's growth path and, consequently, its broader development path—insofar as the latter is premised on core, economic priorities that establish the key terms on which development and reconstruction can be pursued. (p. 37)

GEAR was developed with help from the World Bank. It was drafted and adopted in a process strongly criticized for lack of consultation and debate (Bond, 2000). Not brought before Nedlac, the tripartite structure of business, labor and government, it was declared "non-negotiable" by Minister of Finance Trevor Manuel (Bond, 2000, p. 91). GEAR modeling predicted that by 2000 the economy would be growing by 6%, with 400,000 new jobs created annually (RSA, 1996).

However, it soon became clear that GEAR could not meet its established goals, especially for jobs and consistent growth. Instead of the employment growth of 3% to 4% promised by GEAR, there were annual job losses between 1% to 4% in the late 1990s (Bond, 2000). Growth stood at an average 2.4%. Unemployment grew to 43%, while labor productivity increased and days lost to strikes decreased. The deficit was maintained below 3% through social spending restrictions, despite huge unemployment. Inequality in the already vastly unequal society increased (COSATU, 2000). According to government statistics, black African household income fell 19% between 1995 and 2000 (to $3,714 per year). Over the same period, white household income rose 15% (to $22,600 per year) (Bond, 2004a). The state raised the cost of water and electricity, and people who could not pay for the service were cut off. Access to these and other basic services declined (Bond, Dor, & Ruiters, 2000).

Independent research by COSATU (see Table 1) shows that there were declines in access to electricity and flush toilets for poor South Africans and modest gains in access to other services.

But in the analysis of this data they add (COSATU, 2000),

> But in economic terms, for many households, the gains have been offset by rising unemployment and the resulting fall in income in poor households. Every African family now has some unemployed members. (p. 15)

The National Labor and Economic Development Institute (NALEDI) released a gendered critique of GEAR, which built on the literature of economic gender bias (Orr, Heintz, & Tregenna, 1998). The authors note that references to women and gender are absent in the GEAR policy and that it committed the fallacy of

Table 1. Change in Access to Basic Services 1995–2000

Service	1995	2000	% Change
Formal housing	66%	73%	7%
Electricity for lighting	64%	72%	6%
Electricity for cooking	55%	54%	−1%
Electricity for heating	54%	51%	−3%
Piped water	79%	84%	5%
Flush toilet	57%	56%	−1%

Source: Statistics South Africa (2002).

making invisible women's reproductive and informal economic contributions. In particular, the authors note that the rolling back of state services required by GEAR places an undue, economically invisible (in that it is not calculated) burden as women pick up the slack in their unpaid labor.

Health System Transformation in Postapartheid South Africa

Health system transformation in post-1994 South Africa aimed at redressing historic inequities in access to health services through integrating existing services in the public sector, redirecting toward primary health services delivered through a district-based system, and shifting expenditures toward primary and preventative services away from curative hospital-based services (Stack & Hlela, 2002). South Africa entered negotiations with the apartheid government better prepared in health policy than other policy areas. This was based upon the deep roots of primary health care (PHC) in South Africa, dating back to the early 1950s (Abdool-Karim & Abdool-Karim, 2002). Beginning in the 1980s public health activists organized to address the social and political aspects of health issues under apartheid. As part of the UDF and ANC, groups such as the Progressive Primary Health Care Network explored and drafted alternative health policies.

In the 1994 Reconstruction and Development Programme (RDP), the public health influence is central. In the RDP health is defined through mental, physical, and social aspects, and the document links health back to economic development and other social policy areas. The plan for a district-based system based on Primary Health Care principles (PHC) is outlined in the RDP. The plan also calls for harnessing the activities of both private- and public-sector health care under a national system (ANC, 1992).

In 1997 the ANC, under Minister of Health Dr. N. C. Dlamini Zuma, released the White Paper on Health System Transformation (1997). The objectives of this guiding document are listed in Table 2. The general thrust of these policies developed by progressive public health advocates and expressed in the RDP remained intact in the White Paper.

However, neither the RDP nor the White Paper challenges the private/public split in health services, though the White Paper does lay out the need to reinstate regulations on medical schemes that had been removed in the late 1980s. This led to denial of benefits for those with preexisting conditions, reductions in benefits, and use of the public system to pick up the slack (private patients were shifted to public hospitals when their benefits ran out). Meanwhile, universal national health coverage is now advocated by progressive coalitions and is part of the people's budget platform (People's Budget Campaign, 2003). In part this is a response to the distorting effect of the public/private split, in which private services take up far larger and increasing costs (Benatar, 2004).

Transformation of the health sector was severely constrained by limits on spending imposed by GEAR, as well as the switch to a global budgeting system (akin to the block-grant system in the United States) that puts health in direct competition with other budgets at the provincial level (Stack & Hlela, 2002). Critical here is the fact that at the highest levels of government, the proportion of funds available for health care are limited by debt repayments (Bond, 2004). Thus, the enormous strain on the health system due to HIV/AIDS taxed dwindling resources. South African public hospitals received reduced funding and hiring and wage freezes resulted (Stack & Hlela, 2002). South African policy observers have also noted that the "top-down" GEAR policy replaced a "people-centered" approach, another characteristic of GEAR that constrained health-sector development by limiting input (Willan, 2004).

In South Africa the public health sector competes in various ways with a large private health sector. Figures for 1999 show that R25 billion from medical

Table 2. Objectives of Health Sector Restructuring

- To unify fragmented health services at all levels into a comprehensive and integrated National Health System.
- To promote equity, accessibility and utilization of health services.
- To extend the availability and ensure the appropriateness of health services.
- To develop health promotion activities.
- To develop human resources available to the health sector.
- To foster community participation across the health sector.
- To improve health sector planning and the monitoring of health status and services.

Source: White Paper on Health Sector Transformation (1997).

insurance schemes was spent for 7 to 8 million people receiving care in the private sector, while R24 billion was spent on 33 million in the public sector, which is also responsible for the country's medical training (Benatar, 2004). Private hospitals have thrived in the postapartheid era, draining doctors, nurses, patients and income from the public system. Over the past 30 years, expenditure for private care has grown considerably. In the 1970s, 30% of health expenditure was concentrated in the 20% of the population with insurance. In 2004, 60% of health expenditure went for 18% with insurance (Benatar, 2004). The percentage of South African doctors who work in the private system has grown from 40% in 1970 to over 66% today.

Claims concerning the efficiency of private entities are called into question by the fact that far more money is spent in the private sector providing care for significantly fewer people than is spent in the public sector. As one study puts it (Stack & Hlela, 2002),

> Cost escalation is rampant in the private sector, and the overall level of funding to achieve a package of services is very high. (p. 12)

A key informant in the case study noted these comparisons of procedure costs in the private versus public setting: R16,000 for a cesarean childbirth at a private hospital versus R3,500 at a public hospital; R12,000 for a midwife-assisted birth at a private hospital versus R5,000 at a public one (Mitchell, FM).

An analysis of the 2005 South African budget notes that while public health spending has remained constant, spending in the private sector has soared. As a result, health spending is around 8% of GDP (while it is 5% to 6% for other comparable countries (People's Budget Campaign, 2005).

Despite evidence that shows that private health care has higher costs, South African public hospitals are engaging in various methods to privatize in order to compete with the private sector. These include establishing private wards in public hospitals, allowing private physicians admitting privileges to public facilities, and the contracting out of nonmedical services to private firms (RSA, 2004).

Commenting on the impact to poor South Africans of the current system, Benatar (2004) notes,

> A two-tiered health care system thus continues, with discrimination in access to care on economic grounds replacing the racial discrimination of the past. (p. 88)

Benatar's comment echoes Bonds conclusions in his analysis of GEAR (Bond, 2004a):

> The reality is that South Africa has witnessed the replacement of racial apartheid with what is increasingly referred to as class apartheid—systemic underdevelopment and segregation of the oppressed majority through struc-tured economic, political, legal, and cultural practices. (p. 47)

The impacts of GEAR on health sector development has been to reproduce and intensify inequalities in South Africa on the basis of class instead of race, an extension of the harms it has caused South African workers generally. At the same time, class and race are closely correlated, as are class, race, and the risk of being infected with HIV (UNAIDS, 2004). Beginning in the mid-to-late 1990s, HIV/AIDS and the related TB epidemic became the predominant challenge in the South African public health sector.

The Explosion of HIV/AIDS in Postapartheid South Africa

Before his assassination in 1991, Chris Hani, Spear of the Nation Leader, sent a message to fellow ANC members (Abdool-Karim & Abdool-Karim, 2002):

> Those of us in exile are in the unfortunate situation of being in the areas where the prevalence is high. We cannot afford to allow the AIDS epidemic to ruin the realization of our dreams. Existing statistics indicate that we are still at the beginning of the AIDS epidemic in our country. Unattended, however, this will result in untold damage and suffering by the end of the century. (p. 39)

The HIV/AIDS epidemic exploded in South Africa in the postapartheid period. In 1994 HIV prevalence was estimated at 1%. In the decade that followed, prevalence estimates have been as high as 37% in some areas, with far higher concentrations in particular communities: townships, former rural "homeland" areas, and makeshift shanty towns (UNAIDS, 2004). The southern African region is identified by UNAIDS as the "worst affected sub-region" in the world, and South Africa has the highest number of people living with HIV of any county in the world. Within South Africa, KZN has the highest HIV prevalence among pregnant women, 37.5%, of South Africa's nine provinces based on Department of Health data. Across the Southern African region there are 13 HIV positive women for every 10 HIV positive men, and HIV infection among pregnant South African women has continued to rise each year since 2001 (UNAIDS, 2004).

The conditions for the rapid explosion of the HIV/AIDS epidemic can be traced specifically to apartheid-era policies such as forced removals, lack of housing and services for blacks in urban areas, and the destruction of African families as exemplified by the living situation of mine workers and the prevalence of violence (Marks, 2002). The route of the spread of HIV/AIDS has been traced to labor migration and transportation routes across SSA (Abdool-Karim & Abdool-Karim, 2002). While it is clear that the current government of South Africa inherited the HIV/AIDS epidemic to a large degree, policies since 1994 have exacerbated the conditions for the epidemic and its spread: poverty, inequality, lack of access to basic services and health care, and until recently, lack of antiretroviral treatment for the poor (Willan, 2004).

In 1990 progressive public health activists and ANC members in exile met in Maputo, Mozambique, and drafted the Maputo Statement on HIV/AIDS (Stein & Zwi, 1990). This statement defined HIV/AIDS as a reflection of political, social, economic, and health conditions that required responses that spoke to these conditions as well as health and human rights needs for people living with HIV/AIDS. The document was created with the input of world class scientists, long-term public health practitioners, and exiled political leaders who were witnessing the effects that HIV/AIDS was already having in southern African countries where they resided. The RDP and White Paper on Health Sector Transformation each reflect the aims of the Maputo Statement, and specific means for implementation (RSA, 1997).

> It is recognised that HIV/AIDS cannot be prevented without addressing the socioeconomic factors which underlie its spread. The cause and impact of AIDS extends beyond the health sector, requiring the commitment of and intervention by a sectors–the State, private sector, nongovernmental organisations (NGOs) and community-based organisations (CBOs).
> The implementation of the National AIDS Control Programme focuses on five central objectives:
> To prevent the spread of the epidemic through the promotion of safer sexual behaviour, adequate provision of condoms and control of STDs; to protect and promote the rights of people living with HIV or AIDS by ensuring that discrimination against such people is outlawed; to use the mass media to popularise key prevention concepts and develop life skills education for youth in and out of school; to reduce the personal and social impact of HIV/AIDS through the provision of counselling, care and social support, including social welfare services for persons with HIV/AIDS, their families and the community; and to mobilise and unify local, provincial, national and international resources to prevent and reduce the impact of HIV/AIDS. (p. 35)

In particular, the White Paper specified civil society groups including National AIDS Convention of South Africa (NACOSA) and the National Association of People Living with HIV/AIDS (NAPWA), which would later become the Treatment Action Campaign (TAC). NACOSA was instrumental in the consultative process that developed the first National AIDS Control Program. However, things swiftly fell apart. Public health practitioners and scientists who were close to the process reported being "shut out" (Coovadia, 2002). In 1996 a financial scandal erupted over a musical production (Sarafina II), which had been intended to be a major AIDS prevention piece. In 1997 Virodene was introduced at the highest level of government as a locally discovered AIDS medicine; this turned out to be an industrial solvent and the promoters noncredentialed. From 1997 onward situations further distanced the ANC leadership from earlier aggressive policy on HIV/AIDS and alienated government officials from civil society groups. For example, in 1997, at a session intended to build social dialogue, the

National Health Minister announced that HIV/AIDS would be made notifiable, undermining the individual rights basis upon which earlier, collaboratively developed policy had been based (Schneider, 2002).

In the late 1990s the situation worsened. The Mbeki administration began to deny the existence of a link between HIV and AIDS; created barriers to implementing programs such as Prevention of Mother to Child Transmission (PMTCT) with a single dose of neviripine (a program that was recently said to have eliminated infant HIV infection in the United States); and blocked the use of compulsory licensing and parallel importation of ARVs (Schneider, 2002; Willan 2004). South Africa's right to take advantage of provisions in the TRIPS agreement under the WTO and ignore pharmaceutical company patents on anti-retroviral drugs was challenged in court but upheld (Heywood, 2005; WTO, 2001). Still, the South African government did not utilize the legal right to produce or import cheap generic drugs (Bond, 1999). At the 2000 International AIDS conference held in Durban, South African scientists, many of them former friends and comrades of ANC leaders in the fight against apartheid, signed a declaration of recognition of the biomedical causes of AIDS (Abdool-Karim & Abdool-Karim, 2002). In 2001, when statistics were released that showed huge increases in AIDS-related mortality in South Africa, the government challenged the data as "unprovable" (Willan, 2004).

In 2003 it was estimated that 600 people died of AIDS each day in South Africa (TAC, 2004). In 2005 statistics were released showing a 57% increase in AIDS-related mortality since 2001, including alarming increases in female deaths (from 144 men per 100 women to 77 men per 100 women) (Statistics South Africa, 2005). The role of antiretroviral treatment in a mature epidemic is to save lives, reduce the stigma of the disease, and help prevention efforts by encouraging testing (Irwin et al., 2003). Thus, the contestation over ARV treatment is important to treatment, prevention, education for HIV/AIDS. Table 3 provides a summary of the history of government response to HIV/AIDS and contestation since 1990.

The struggle for HIV/AIDS treatment in South Africa is led by the Treatment Action Campaign (TAC) COSATU coalition, and is part of a broader independent left movement (Bond, 2005). HIV/AIDS treatment has been demanded as part of a package of policies that includes investment in public services including health, a basic income grant, and new policies for jobs creation (Bond, 2005). The TAC has been mentored by veteran U.S. and European AIDS activists such as ACT-UP and the Treatment Action Group (Epstein, 1996). These groups were vital in setting a research agenda and provided a model for how lay people could become involved in scientific agenda setting. Differences between the two movements are the class-based politics in South Africa versus identity politics in the U.S.-based movement (Epstein, 1996; Schneider, 2002). The TAC is led by former antiapartheid activists, and includes campaigns to monitor public sector health services and a health care workers campaign. The TAC and the AIDS

Table 3. Key Events in South African AIDS Policy

1990	Maputo Statement drafted
1994	NACOSA launched
1996	National HIV/AIDS STD program launched
1996	*Sarafina II* musical criticized
1997	Virodene announced
1997	AIDS made notifiable by the Minister of Health
1998-99	AZT questioned
1999	TAC launched from NAPWA to fight for AIDS treatment
2000	Launch of National AIDS Council by the government, excluding activists and scientists
2000	Cause of AIDS questioned by the presidency; Durban Declaration by scientists
2001	Use of ARVs in the public sector rejected by the Ministry of Health
2001	Delays in implementation of PMTCT by Ministry of Health
2001	Mortality statistics questioned by the presidency
2002	TAC wins court case to extend PMTCT; government releases statement that policy will go on the assumption that HIV causes AIDS, and admits usefulness of ARVs and releases plan to provide them to rape victims for post-exposure prophylaxis
2003[a]	Government releases plans to provide ARVs in the public sector
2003	Minister of Health expresses reluctance to roll out ARVs; president denies extent of epidemic
2004	ARV treatment in the public sector commences
2004	TAC renews campaign to fight for swifter treatment implementation

[a]Events listed after 2003 occurred after the case study used in this book.
Sources: Schneider (2002), Willan (2004), Abdool-Karim & Abdool-Karim (2002).

Law Project are largely credited in South Africa with pushing ANC policy. Civil disobedience, on the eve of the countries third national election, posed a threat to the ANC's political base (Willan, 2004).

In November 2003, on the eve of South Africa's third national election, the ANC approved a national HIV/AIDS treatment plan that would supply ARVs through the public health system (RSA, 2003a).[3] This followed a year of increasing TAC protest, both in South Africa and internationally, which culminated in planned civil disobedience actions in March of 2003, during which AIDS activists and people living with HIV/AIDS were sprayed with hoses and beaten by police (Willan, 2004). However, the plan has not been enacted, key money has not been allocated, and government officials have made statements that seemingly detract from commitment to the plan. Money for the new AIDS plan represented the bulk of health sector spending in the new budget (Idasa, 2004). While the plan contains expenditures to strengthen the national health system, since the money is "ring-fenced" in the budget, failure to enact will equal a real shortfall to the public health system (People's Budget Campaign, 2003).

In 2004 another round of civil disobedience was planned to protest the slow pace of implementation of the 2003 AIDS plan. As retired Constitutional Court Judge Edwin Cameron notes (Willan, 2004), "there is still a dualism between governmental statement and action." In September 2003 President Mbeki publicly stated, "Personally, I don't know anyone who has died of AIDS. I really honestly don't" (Slevin, 2003).

Many South Africans have written about the Mbeki/ANC denial of HIV/AIDS. Some observers noted that early lack of political will might be explained in part by the unforeseen difficulties in implementing ambitious health sector reform (Schneider & Stein, 2001). Others associated attitudes of denial with healthy suspicion of Western medicine based on apartheid-era experiences (there is an often-repeated story that the apartheid government planned to deliberately infect Africans with HIV/AIDS or poison them with medicines) (Schneider & Fassin, 2002). Distrust of Western approaches to health and stereotypes of Africans have also been held up as the reason that Mbeki has persisted in linking HIV/AIDS with poverty and poor nutrition, and resisting claims that stigmatize Africans as more "at risk" than others. Others, including nurses in the case study that follows, associate denial with the government not wanting to pay to fight HIV/AIDS. While it is not possible to know definitively why Mbeki's denial took root or has been so strong, the impacts are more clear.

The contestation over AIDS policy and government inaction has resulted in misinformation generated by trusted leadership and a fissure in the public health community. Messages about the toxicity of AIDS drugs and the doubtful motives of Western scientists have coexisted with government statements about

---

[3] This occurred after the case study that is presented in this book.

how AIDS is really caused by poverty and poor nutrition—a position that converges with the public health perspective. Public health practitioners who, in the context of a mature epidemic, must reconcile the idea of HIV prevention with the secondary prevention that can be achieved from antiretroviral drugs, are in the position of "medicalizing" a public health issue with vast political and social dimensions. This situation threatens the effectiveness of prevention and treatment efforts; when misinformation and stigma prevails, people do not seek testing and counseling that opens the door to prevention and treatment (Marais, 1999; Schneider & Fassin, 2003).

On the ground, government denial and failure to implement policies meant that while people became infected, sick, and died, these facts were met with inadequate government response. Newspaper reports revealed the extent of the impacts to the community: money spent on funerals threatened families survival; many reported attending funerals every weekend; a crisis due to lack of burial space was predicted (Moore, 2003). Further, denial and stigma were important barriers to prevention at the community level. Following the International AIDS Conference in Durban in 2000, a woman who publicly revealed her status was later stoned to death when she returned home to her village (South African Press Association [SAPA], 2001). My own experiences in South Africa confirmed the phenomena of denial and stigma. At a conference at the university in Durban, I met community home-based care volunteers from rural KwaZulu-Natal, who had no problem revealing that they were HIV positive, but told me they could not tell anyone in their community, not even their families or other AIDS program volunteers due to stigma.

CHAPTER CONCLUSION

In 1994 South Africa achieved freedom from apartheid and held its first democratic elections. Abandoning years of ANC socialist rhetoric, the newly elected ANC leaders responded to the policy context of structural adjustment in Africa and the victory of market-based capitalism after the fall of the Berlin wall, by adopting neoliberal policies embodied in the GEAR program. This has led to specific harms to the working class, increases in entrenched inequality, and wage and spending freezes on health services. These were particularly harmful because of the explosion of HIV/AIDS; and harmful effects were multiplied by government misinformation about HIV/AIDS and failure to adopt decisive, strong policies that drew on the resources of South Africa for public health, research, and community organizing.

1. The replacement of the RDP document with GEAR marked a postapartheid shift toward neoliberal policies.
2. Top-down GEAR policies increased unemployment, inequality, and reduced democratic input.

3. GEAR policies constrained postapartheid health sector transformation and exacerbated the conditions for the explosion of HIV/AIDS.
4. The dynamics of government denial of HIV/AIDS also allowed the epidemic to worsen and spread denial and misinformation in the community.

Despite the fact that the victory over apartheid was led in part by a militant politicized labor movement, labor faced immediate challenges in the post-apartheid era. Most serious, the 1996 GEAR policy led to massive job losses that left the working class struggling. Organized Labor also struggled to develop a program and response to the challenges of globalization. This was complicated by the fact that struggle occurred within what had been a cohesive left wing during the struggle against apartheid. Social issues such as women's position and the HIV/AIDS epidemic took a back seat to basic survival issues. Further, many observers note that organized labor in South Africa was significantly weakened in the postapartheid era, as strong leaders left for leadership roles in government. The relative weakness of labor in this period influences the development of a labor/work-environment approach to health. As the working class struggles over basic issues, larger social questions take a back seat.

CHAPTER 3

❦

The Work Environment of Nurses

This chapter provides background on the history of nursing in South Africa, as well as brief exploration of how to understand this history from a work environment perspective.

THEORY OF THE WORK ENVIRONMENT

How is occupational illness determined by the political, social, and industry context in health care?

Given that what happens in the workplace is a reflection of the larger political economy—the relative power of workers, government, and companies—the rise of privatization and commodification of care is determinative of the health care work environment and the quality of care that is provided. Nursing has historically been affected by health care industry shifts that have exploited race and gender issues. For example, the rise of hospital-based care in the United States created a need for nurses, which was met in part by creating schools of nursing attached to hospitals to supply student nurses, and in part by hiring nurses for shift work. Both phenomena (in addition to the wartime need for nurses) drew working class women into the ranks of nursing, which previously had been reserved for the middle class. Nurses' position in the hospital hierarchy, along with the fact that it is traditionally women's work, has kept wages lower, and divisions among nurses along racial lines have created the basis for divisions among nurses, where women of color have performed the least attractive jobs and filled the most undesirable shifts (Melosch, 1982). Currently nurses around the world face a work environment characterized by increasing workloads and decreasing public investment.

Wooding and Levenstein (1999) developed a theory of work environment for advanced industrial societies that places management's control of the workplace at the center of occupational health. Their model posits that "the key relationship for understanding the work environment is a 'triangle' of control representing management's dominance of workplace, workers, and any potential hazards" (p. 13). The central point of this theory is that occupational health is determined by how power is distributed in the workplace, and this in turn depends on the political and economic context of production. Another key aspect of this theory is that what happens at the "point of production" determines social relations and policy.

But the triangle of control must be interpreted slightly differently in analyzing the worksite hazards faced by service-sector workers. For service workers, it is more useful to think about the "point of consumption," which refers to work environments in which the relationship between the worker and the public is a key component of the service produced. The relationship may also affect the injury experience of service workers. Needlestick and back injuries in health care and violence in retail and social services are examples of service industry injuries that have gained attention over the period in which service-sector employment has increased (Slattery, 1998; United States Department of Labor [USDOL], 1996). During the 1990s, a decline in reported occupational injuries and illnesses was attributed by some to safer conditions in service-sector employment (compared with other sectors) or to the success of existing policies (Brown, 2007). However, new research indicates that hazards in service-sector jobs—such as violence, ergonomic risks, and indoor air quality (including ETS)—may go unidentified and unreported when occupational health risks are undetected by such traditional surveillance methods as OSHA (Occupational Safety and Health Administration) logs and labor-management health and safety committees (Azaroff et al., 2002).

In the context of neoliberal globalization, the work environment may be characterized by a "race to the bottom." Many researchers have commented on how the globalized economy puts the most desperate workers at a disadvantage. Brown (2004) looks at how the search for the cheapest labor in the least regulated environments has led to increased vulnerability of the workforce. Loewenson (1999) illustrates how southern African women, as the least powerful group, are disproportionately affected by worsening conditions of work.

The history of nursing is bifurcated between the "call" to care, heavily influenced by religious institutions and prescriptions about women's social role, and the development of an industry reliant on wage labor. Melosch (1982) describes the history of nursing in the United States as "more than a story of professionalization, nursing history is the story of women workers experience in a rationalizing service industry" (p. 7). This statement could be extended to apply to HCW in the context of a global move toward market-based health care. As providers of care in a privatizing environment, women in particular face devaluing of their work and increased burdens at home as care costs are externalized (Turshen, 1999). Brannon (1994) has characterized the "intensification" of the health care work environment in the United States. Hospitals seeking to compete in the managed environment seek work-organization solutions to short-staffing brought on by cuts in labor costs. Patient acuity in the hospital increases as services for the less sick are delivered outpatient.

Similarly, in South Africa, as hospitals became overcrowded with HIV/AIDS patients, a policy of home-based, palliative care was adopted (Akintola, 2004). This has intensified the existing burden of care that women experience, and led to informalization of health care that is characterized by an increased unpaid burden to women, and shifted the hazards of this work (occupational exposure to HIV/AIDS and stress) into the home. Privatization has decreased access to health care throughout southern Africa and led to increased burdens on women and disinvestment in the work environment. (Turshen, 1999).

Marks (1994) describes the history of the hospital work environment for nurses in South Africa through the tensions of race/class divisions among female health workers. Conditions were always worse for black nurses in South Africa's public-sector hospitals. Marks describes how the need for a workforce that would accept lower pay won out over apartheid restrictions about who could nurse whom (i.e., the taboo against black hands on white bodies). Black nurses came to predominate at bedside in public-sector hospitals because they could be paid two thirds of what white nurses earned, were grateful for any employment, and would accept poor working conditions. As black women, nurses' experience of occupational risk was determined by their lack of power in the workplace. Ironically, as one of the only professions open to Africans, male or female, in the colonial/apartheid eras, African nurses had an elevated social position outside of the workplace (Mashaba, 1995).

VIEWS ON THE AFRICAN/SOUTH AFRICAN HIV/AIDS EPIDEMIC

Why has South Africa suffered such a devastating impact from HIV/AIDS?

The South African HIV/AIDS epidemic has a complex set of causes that can be understood from a variety of levels (from biomedical to macro). The progressive public health understanding of the HIV/AIDS epidemic in South Africa connects it to the history of colonial exploitation and structural adjustment, and sees the epidemic that disproportionately affects poor, female Africans as a form of "structural violence." In South Africa, migrant labor and transportation routes spurred the spread of HIV/AIDS, while the postapartheid ANC government's slowness in addressing the disease facilitated its explosion.

Barnett and Whiteside (2002) developed a framework that describes the levels of causation of HIV/AIDS, which runs from the structural, macrolevel to the biological dynamics of the organism in the human body. Their framework captures the complexity of factors that contribute to an HIV/AIDS epidemic, as well as the variety of interventions that may be conceived. At the most proximate levels, AIDS is caused by HIV infection that is determined by biomedical factors. These factors can only occur in the presence of exposure, which is determined by behavior (sexual, drug use). Behavior in turn has socioeconomic determinants or associations, and these occur within a broader context that the authors refer to through wealth, income distribution, governance, and so forth. Interventions are only noted for biomedical and behavioral levels.

Barnett and Whiteside use this framework in a comparison of the epidemic in six countries, and conclude that social cohesion can explain the unequal impact of HIV/AIDS. The work of Wilkinson (2002) shows that countries with higher levels of income inequality experience worse health outcomes. The social cohesion theory posits that this is due to the harmful effects of hierarchy on social relations. Mutaner and Lynch (2002) have criticized Wilkinson for ignoring class structure and class formation, and argue that health inequalities originate in class interests and the unequal distribution of power and control.

Farmer (1999) posits that the cause of global disparities of HIV/AIDS is rooted in what he terms "structural violence." By this he means a system that is overtly harmful. In this view, the HIV/AIDS epidemic in Africa is directly linked to the history of colonialism and exploitation, current debt repayment, and lack of bargaining power over international prices for raw materials—in short, all the factors that made and have kept Africa poor despite its wealth and resources and the hard work of its people. Marks (2002) and Benatar (2002) describe the link between global inequality and the spread of AIDS. Rowden (2004) argues that the IMF focuses on policies that keep inflation low; ties the hands of developing countries, who cannot increase health spending due to policies aimed at inflation; and conditionalities that punish policy change with withdrawal of financial support.

Zierler and Krieger make a similar argument, starting from the observation that "social inequalities lie at the heart of risk of HIV infection among women living in poor countries and among poor women living in wealthy countries" (Zierler & Krieger, 1998). They develop their perspective by noting that while literature and research on women and HIV focuses on biomedical, lifestyle, and psychological theories of disease causation, social frameworks (including feminist, political economy, ecosocial theory and human rights) facilitate a more accurate understanding of HIV risk. Zierler and Krieger's approach seems to be supported by the direction of the HIV/AIDS pandemic since the time of their article, as women of color worldwide have become a disproportionate burden of HIV/AIDS.

Basu (2004) makes the link between intervention and attribution of cause by arguing that the overwhelming concern with sexual behavior change and the health-belief model in AIDS prevention interventions leads to false assumptions.

> Given that the top epidemiological predictor for HIV infection around the world is not "risk behavior" but rather a low income level, those most vulnerable to infection will not benefit from a model focused on

"education"—a model that assumes people in poverty have the agency to control the circumstances of their lives, even in the context of gender inequality or in environments without income opportunities other than trading sex for money. (p. 156)

The focus of the President's Emergency Plan for AIDS Relief (PEPFAR, the plan released by President Bush in 2003 to fight global AIDS) on programs that promote abstinence, do not support abortion, and provide education that has not been shown to affect the spread of AIDS is criticized by Basu and others. Basu (2004) notes that it is not sex per se that leads to HIV/AIDS, but the context of sex. Benatar (2001) terms the failure and dismay over international efforts to address HIV/AIDS in the developing world "naïve" given the obvious role of poverty and the forces that perpetuate it on the epidemic, and the lack of scope of interventions.

Harrison, Wilkinson, Lurie, Connoly, and Abdool-Karim (1998) studied the spread of HIV/AIDS and the routes of labor migration in Africa/South Africa. The Southern African Migration Project (SAMP; Crush, Peberdy, & Williams, 2006) found strong associations between trucking routes and the spread of HIV/AIDS in Africa, as well as links to the communities of origin.[1] Abdool-Karim and Abdool-Karim (2002) note that transportation routes in sub–Saharan Africa also contribute to disease spread. These correlations explain how South Africa, as the destination of African migrants and main pipeline in the flow of goods, came to suffer among the worst HIV/AIDS epidemics as a direct outcome of its economic advantage; they describe the specific "context of sex" that has fostered the spread of HIV/AIDS in Africa. There is a historical precedent for the disease/ work-pattern link. In 1949 Kark argued that in relation to South Africa's rampant syphilis epidemic, the migrant labor system on which South Africa's industrial-ization was premised was perhaps the single most important cause of ill-health (Kark, 2002). Williams and Campbell (1996) describe the occupational link further, noting that the excellent hospitals provided for miners did nothing to treat the illnesses that took hold after they returned home, effectively externalizing the costs of diseases that were linked to the situation of migrants.

Zwi and Cabral (1991) argued that a new term, "high risk situations," should be employed to understand the set of factors that increase vulnerability to HIV/AIDS, including the social, economic, and political forces that place groups at high risk. Marks (2002) notes that this criteria helps to explain why HIV/AIDS has been so devastating in South Africa given the history of exploitation, social disruption, and violence.

Marais (1999) and others (Adelzadeh, 1996; Bond, 2000; Saul, 2001) chronicled the failure of the postapartheid ANC-led government to effectively

---

[1] HIV/AIDS spreads through sex workers on migrant routes, but is also brought to stable communities of origin on visits home.

address HIV/AIDS, among other social issues. In particular, early failures to implement prevention policies developed before the first democratic elections in 1994; failures to involve local scientists and public health activists; government misinformation about HIV/AIDS treatment; and failure to introduce and then to implement treatment policies have been identified as factors that fueled the spread of HIV/AIDS. In addition, post-1994 policies that increased poverty and inequality have also been identified as contributing to the spread and impacts of the epidemic (Benatar, 2004).

Social movements are another factor that influenced the spread of HIV/AIDS and public and medical response to the disease. Beginning in the 1980s, Act-Up and the Treatment Action Group engaged in a range of activities fought for the rights and for treatment for HIV/AIDS when it was viewed as a primarily gay disease. Epstein (1996) describes how these movements used science literacy to successfully involve themselves in a highly technical policy process and how individuals in Europe and the United States became mentors to AIDS activists in South Africa. Parker (2003) has reviewed how social movements for treatment led by people living with HIV/AIDS have altered the course of epidemics by securing treatment. For example, Brazil adopted universal access to ARV treatment in the context of a popular social movement and the political ambitions of a health ministry figure who, despite alliances to neoliberal positions, wanted a feather in his cap in a run for political office. Brazil implemented free universal access to ARV treatment in the public sector, and its prevalence rates have been stable since the early 1990s. Friedman and Mottiar (2004) describe how the social movement for HIV/AIDS treatment in South Africa—the Treatment Action Campaign—had intimate ties to the antiapartheid struggle historically and has ties to the anti-neoliberal struggle contemporarily. Friedman and Mottiar (2004) describe the precarious position of the TAC as a movement that focuses specifically on the fight for treatment and the medical aspects of HIV/AIDS, and that at times supports the range of public health and development issues that relate to provision of treatment and the spread of disease.

Much of the activism related to the inequalities of HIV/AIDS has focused on treatment. Pharmaceutical companies have gained huge profits from AIDS medicines and gone to great lengths to protect these profits (Davis & Fort, 2004). Davis and Fort (2004) describe how trade rules have protected patent holders, but also provided opportunities for the production and importation of generic drugs. However, recent trade negotiations have focused on bilateral agreements that bypass "TRIPS loopholes"[2] (Shaffer & Brenner, 2004).

---

[2]Trade-Related Aspects of Intellectual Property Rights (TRIPS) loopholes were upheld at the 2001 round of trade talks convened by the WTO at Doha. The Declaration on the TRIPS agreement and public health supports the right for developing counties to produce or import generic medicines, even if these are under existing patent.

Since 2000 there has been a sea of change in attitudes toward HIV/AIDS treatment in the developing world. The goal of providing ARV treatment for the world's poor is now socially acceptable and involves many donor efforts (Irwin et al., 2003). D'Adesky (2004) evaluates the progress of donor efforts and notes areas of progress and impediments. Serious impediments to supplying treatment are shortages of health care workers (Chen et al., 2004a); underfunded programs (McCoy et al., 2005); macroeconomic constraints due to IMF conditionalities that hamper governments' ability to invest in health or absorb donations (Rowden, 2004); and barriers to generic drug production (Davis & Fort, 2004). In South Africa there has been a persistent struggle between civil society and government over providing HIV/AIDS treatment. Willan (2004) describes how, on the one hand, international pressure has pushed the ANC-led government to enact national ARV treatment policy. On the other hand, international pressures over patents and generic production have influenced how treatment policy is developed (D'Adesky, 2004).

BRAIN DRAIN AND THE GLOBAL NURSING SHORTAGE

What is the connection between nursing shortages in various countries in the developed and developing world?

Nursing shortages aren't new, but their global scope is a more recent development. Brain drain from south to north, developing to developed countries, exacerbates shortages in places where HCWs are badly needed. This issue has recently received policy attention from a variety of perspectives, particularly given the global HIV/AIDS pandemic, but a workers' rights focus is lacking in the mainstream response.

Nursing shortages were created along with the hospital-based system of care that created the bulk of nursing jobs. Melosch (1982) dates the first nursing shortage in contemporary nursing history to 1948 and the postwar hospital expansion in the United States. In their discussion of the link between nurse salaries and labor supply, Chihaa and Link (2003) describe the ebb and flow of the U.S. shortage of nurses since the 1970s. They note that the most recent shortage of nurses, beginning in the mid-to-late 1990s, differed from previous shortages because it is (a) international in scope and (b) related to the impacts of health-sector changes, which have led to mandatory overtime, intentional short-staffing, and reductions in ancillary services.

Nursing shortages in South Africa also have a long history. Marks (1994) describes how shortages of white nurses in the public sector were engineered through pay differentials between private and public-sector nursing. Despite strict apartheid policy that dictated nurses and patients must be of the same race, economic policy ensured that black nurses would fill the numerous ranks of the lower rungs of nursing. A "shortage" of white nurses necessitated an inflow of those who would settle for lower pay and worse conditions of work.

During the 1990s the issue of the impact of health reforms on health workers was examined under the rubric of "human resources for health." Martinez and Martineau (1998), researchers with World Bank affiliations, assess that nurses have borne the brunt of health reforms in the developing world, which have shrunk health budgets while demanding quality reforms. They recommend that the role of HR be strengthened to repair and ameliorate impacts to nurses. Their call for "human resources for health for the new millennium" linked the need for strong workforces to meeting population health goals and contributed to an increase in the study of health workers in the developing world.

There is a growing body of evidence that shows how nursing shortages in developing countries are linked to the brain drain of skilled health workers from south to north, and how this situation is exacerbated by HIV/AIDS (Padarath, Chamberlain, McCoy, Ntuli, Rowson, & Loewenson, 2003). Once programs to treat HIV/AIDS in poor countries became the goal of global initiatives, it was swiftly recognized that health care worker shortages posed a grave threat to the success of such programs. But, despite broad agreement, there remain significant differences in analysis and approach to the issues of shortages. For example, these range from a Physicians for Human Rights (PHR, 2004) focus on human rights and criticisms of the role of the IMF and World Bank; to USAID (Huddart & Picazo, 2003) recommendations that neoliberal reforms must have an eye on HR issues; to the Joint Learning Initiatives (JLI, 2004) overt concern with the Millennium Development Goal effort, focus on the human resource management side, and omission of the mention of trade unions as a potential partner in change efforts. The Equinet Africa brief (Padarath et al., 2003) looks in-depth at the factors that are pushing and pulling southern African HCW toward migration for better pay and working conditions. Padarath et al. (2003) describe the global picture as a "global conveyer belt," which pulls health care workers from rural to urban areas regionally, and from south to north globally. Notably, as the economic powerhouse of its region, South Africa has both the highest population density of HCW and the greatest number out-migrating (JLI, 2004).

It is worth noting here that the "push-pull" framework for understanding labor migration has been criticized for not taking into account the manner in which immigration and economic policies have been predicated on migration. Under push-pull, poor working and economic conditions in the home country push migrants to seek work abroad, while need and better pay and conditions pull migrants toward receiving countries. But this model does not sufficiently identify the intent with which these situations arise. For example, in the Philippines, an excess of nurses are deliberately trained for the purpose of export to the United States. This creates a flow of wealth back to the home economy, facilitates insufficient training of U.S. nurses, hinders labor solidarity, and provides a lower cost investment in training and education. Building on the work of Saskia Sassen

(1990), Grace Chang charges that "first world countries make deliberate economic interventions to facilitate their continued extraction of third world resources, including and especially people" (Chang, 2000).

Since 2003 the international policy response to the issues of health care worker shortages—brain drain—retention of health care workforce in developing countries, and shortages in rural areas, has increased substantially. In 2006 the WHO released its plan, "Treat, Train and Retain," to address health care worker shortages in countries that face a severe epidemic of HIV/AIDS (WHO, 2006). A new member-based coalition, the Global Health Worker Alliance, and been launched within the WHO, coordinating the efforts to address the complex issues facing countries looking to solve the complex of problems that contribute to health care worker shortages. Many labor organizations have passed resolutions calling for an end to recruiting health workers away from countries suffering from HIV/AIDS epidemics, and for improvements to working conditions in developed counties to reduce need (Reilly, 2003).

NURSES, HIV/AIDS,
AND OCCUPATIONAL HEALTH

*How have the issues of nurses, HIV/AIDS, and
occupational health been researched for Africa?*

Like other occupational health issues, the study of needlestick injuries has led to different preventive measures, including the focus on personal protective equipment (gloves, safe devices, needle disposal boxes). Some researches have also looked at the population level to determine the circumstances that make needlestick injuries more likely. More than a decade of research on needlestick injuries in the United States has shown that working conditions play an important role in risk and prevention of sharps injuries. There are few Africa-based investigations of nurses occupational health; those that exist show serious problems related to HIV/AIDS, especially stress and occupational exposure to blood. A unique union-based project in South Africa has explored how the HIV/AIDS-related threats to nurses' safety at work could be at the center of shop-floor activism that might lead to developing a dynamic "culture of care" in the South African health sector.

The emergence of the HIV/AIDS epidemic made needlestick injuries among health care workers an important area of study. Most studies were done in the United States. Over the years, vast amounts of research have looked at the prevalence of needlesticks, what types of injuries are the most dangerous, and what procedures commonly result in injury. Good data resulted in the introduction of policies and safer equipment (Clarke, Sloane, & Aiken, 2003).

In a 1997 critical review of the literature, Hanrahan and Reutter concluded that the knowledge base about how to prevent injuries had changed the type but not the number of injuries. They warned that additional studies of organizational and behavioral factors were necessary to understand why needlesticks occurred in order to prevent them. In 1998 Aiken et al. found that needlesticks were unreported three fourths of the time, and that recapping[3] and temporary work assignments were significantly associated with injuries. Based on their data, they speculated that downsizing and deprofessionalization of nursing contributed to needlestick injuries. In a 2002 follow-up to this study, Clarke et al. compared injury data with measures of organizational factors and found that the likelihood of injury was three times greater in hospitals with organizational features related to a poor work environment. Nurses who worked on units with low nurse staffing and high emotional exhaustion had twice the risk of suffering a needlestick compared with nurses who worked on units that lacked these characteristics. Overall, they found that needlestick injuries, far from occurring at random, were significantly associated with hospital units that exhibited poor working con- ditions, particularly short-staffing.

The conclusions of Clarke and colleagues show that context, the work environ- ment, has a detrimental effect on worker health. In particular, they identify low staffing and burn-out as culprits. Based on the work of Clarke et al., South African public-sector hospital nurses might be expected to have higher rates of injuries because of the impacts of HIV/AIDS (burn-out) and the impacts of neoliberal policies (short-staffing). The authors suggest that needlestick injuries might serve as a proxy for a broad range of safety and quality issues due to this association with the work environment conditions (Clarke et al., 2002, p. 1119). Thus, their work supports the idea that understanding the context of needlestick injuries can yield information about building a healthier, safer work environment that goes beyond the specifics of the safer use of sharps and needles.

Horsman and Sheeran's 1995 review of the literature on HCW and HIV/AIDS predicted Aiken, Sloane, and Klocinski's (1997) finding that overwork and under- staffing increased the risk of accidental exposure. Of additional interest to this study is their finding that health reform impacted negatively on the quality of care that HCW could deliver and that HCW felt undervalued and stigmatized in their work with PLWA.

There are few specific studies of HCW workplace exposure to HIV/AIDS in Africa, despite the high prevalence of the disease. An article by Sagoe-Moses, Pearson, Perry, and Jagger (2001) noted that while 70% of the world's cases of AIDS are from sub-Saharan Africa, only 4% of needlesticks are reported from there. A Gumodoka, Farot, Berege, and Dolmaus 1997 study of HCW in Tanzania found that 9% of 623 nurses surveyed reported a needlestick during the week proceeding the interview, and that basic resources for safe protocols such as blood and running water were often lacking. An Ofili, Asuzu, and Okojie 2003

[3] The practice of placing a used syringe back into its cap.

study of HCW in Nigeria found similar problems with frequent injuries and lack of basic equipment.

In South Africa, Unger (2002) (in a study discussed at length in the preliminary studies portion of this review) found that needlesticks were common, most injuries not reported, absences and stress were common, and that due to the high prevalence setting and frequent needlesticks, many nurses fatalistically assumed that they had HIV/AIDS. Gounden and Moodley's (2000) study of 265 employees of the obstetrics department at Durban, KZN's largest teaching hospital, found that 13% had had a blood exposure in the previous year. And though a high number had taken advantage of the availability of PEP for their injury, a high proportion discontinued the treatment due to drug side effects.

In southern Africa, where there is a high prevalence of HIV in the community in general, and where women have an elevated risk (see Box 1), another important question is how many health care workers are already HIV positive. A review by Ncayiyana (2004) and research by Shisana, Hall, Maluleke, Chaureau, and Schwabe (2004) shows that prevalence of HIV among HCW is similar to that of the community at large, and that the loss of HCW to HIV/AIDS could pose a significant problem to providing care and treatment in the public and private health systems. Younger African workers were found to be at the greatest risk, posing a serious threat to the next generation of nurses.

What do nurses themselves have to contribute? It has been demonstrated that nurses' active involvement in policymaking and implementation improves the quality of policies to promote worker and patient's health. In Bostwana, Phaladze (2003) found that nurses were only minimally involved in the policy process, despite the fact that their frontline experiences as caregivers and managers provided a wealth of information pertinent to policy.

The Health Workers for Change Initiative (HWFCI) (Fonn & Xaba, 2001) became a World Health Organization (WHO) model for empowering nurses in the effort to improve patient care. Here, issues that faced primarily female staff and female patients (gender issues) were looked at alongside resource and working condition issues (labor issues). This project introduced gender as a key parameter for understanding nurses' performance, attitudes, and constraints at work in the South African context. This project was based on a basic labor/ work-environment principle: that nurses understanding and actions play an important role in workplace change and quality patient care.

A joint project of the Industrial Health Research Group (IHRG), the South Africa Municipal Workers Union (SAMWU), and the Municipal Services Project (MSP) (McDonald & Ruiters, 2005) took a similar approach to the HWFCI, but rooted the activity within the municipal nurses labor union (SAMWU), a worker health and safety NGO (IHRG), and a research project devoted to looking at the impacts of privatization of public services (MSP). This project, "Who Cares for Health Care Workers?" relied on 32 nurse trade-union members as participant researchers. This project found that employers failed to live up to obligations to

Box 1: Women's Burdens and the HIV/AIDS Epidemic

As is the case in other countries, nurses in South Africa are predominantly female (93% in South Africa, 93% in KZN province, 94% in this study).* Nurses' risks and burdens are characterized and exacerbated by gender inequalities.

Women's risks of HIV/AIDS:
- In 2005 young women (15–24 years) in South Africa were four times more likely to be HIV infected than young men; prevalence among young women was 17% compared with 4.4% among young men.**

Women's role in home-based care:
- As the state is no longer able to provide sufficient health care to the poor, this caring role shifts to the communities and homes and, in particular, to women.
- Additional burdens frequently mean that women and girls leave work and school to care for the sick at home.
- This additional burden on women—largely unrecognized and unremunerated—enables the state to renege on its responsibility of providing health care to citizens and limits women's opportunities to realize their rights.
- The government stipend for accredited caregivers is low (R1,000/ month) and very difficult to access.

Women's issues in the labor market:
- Informalization of their work role as care shifts from hospital to community.
- Problems with staffing rural health are exacerbated because women face more impediments to a migrant lifestyle.
- Under neoliberal policies, work that is traditionally female (i.e., nursing and community care) is typically not recognized, and as such pressure to scale back on such services is greater, thereby aggravating the poor working conditions for nurses, women's positions of inequality, and the health care crisis.

Nurses experience a double burden of poor working conditions at work, and then expectations of being caregivers at home, with little support or recognition.

---

*South African Nursing Council, SANC Geographical distribution 2005. Available from: http://www.sanc.co.za/stats/stat2005/distribution%202005xls.htm
**UNAIDS, Epidemic Update 2006.

provide healthy and safe workplaces, but also that nurses add a role in a culture of neglect, acceptance, and individualization of problems (McDonald & Ruiters, 2005). Because of the participatory model, specifically because the people identifying these problems were also those who could change them, there was a clear path from research to activism. In the words of the final report,

> As activist investigators, the participant researchers in this programme not only explored the prevailing attitudes, behaviours, and practices of OH&S but, in doing so, also began to challenge the silence and neglect that characterizes that cultures. (p. 2)

While South Africa has very good occupational health policy on paper, Myers and Macun (1989) point out that there has been a historic disconnect between the activism of black trade unions and the development of OHS policy. Policy development was technical progress, and most gains came under the guise of segregated unions or the apartheid governments attempt to appease militant unionists beginning in the late 1970s. The Who Cares for Health Care Workers? project speaks to the situation in which OHS policy has been divorced from shop-floor activism (especially in health care, with its legacy of nurse socialization) and paves a path to remedy it.

In the next section I turn to how the political economy of postapartheid South Africa, health-sector transformation, and HIV/AIDS impacted on nurses' occupational health through a case study of three provincial hospitals in KZN.

CHAPTER 4

℃ ℘

Case Study Setting:
Three Public Hospitals in
KwaZulu-Natal, South Africa

INTRODUCTION

In the preceding chapters I described how structural adjustment influenced health policy in sub-Saharan Africa and South Africa following independence from colonialism and apartheid rule. I also examined how, tragically, the HIV/AIDS epidemic exploded during this same time period, placing additional strains on health systems and health workers. In the case study that begins with this chapter, I examine in detail how these forces coalesce and shape the working conditions of public-hospital nurses in KwaZulu-Natal, South Africa. To review, theory of the work environment views occupational health as a direct outcome of the power relations that play out in the workplace through management's control over occupational hazards. Here, I use the lens of occupational health as a means to understand how these twin forces—neoliberal globalization and the South African HIV/AIDS epidemic—impact on nurses in their specific workplace setting.

Before embarking on this case study, it is useful to restate and clarify a few points about nurses' occupational risk of HIV/AIDS, because they are so important to what follows. Most nurses are women, and women are disproportionately infected by HIV in South Africa, shown by prevalence and mortality estimates (SSA, 2004; UNAIDS, 2004). In early 2003 there was no treatment available to health care workers and patients in the public sector, and caps on benefits from many private Medical Aide schemes precluded their use to pay for antiretroviral treatment.[1] While research from 2002 found that the majority of Aide schemes (85%) had adequate coverage for ARVs, and 15% had minimal coverage or coverage that was tied to an individual's medical savings account, comments from

---

[1] In November 2003 a program to provide universal access to ARVs through the public health sector was passed.

some nurses and managers indicated that nurses were not using private plans for ARV treatment. They suggested that available plans may have been inadequate, or that nurses' reluctance to be tested affected their uptake of covered benefits. Since 2004 all plans were required to have sufficient ARV coverage by law (Connelly, 2005).

Antiretroviral medicines were available for nurses through their employer only if they could prove that they were infected at work; this was a very tricky issue. The case for workplace infection was established by an HIV test (called voluntary counseling and testing or VCT in South Africa) after a needlestick or other blood exposure. If a nurse is determined to be HIV positive at the time of this test, no compensation coverage is available. Thus, a nurse who was already infected at work through a past exposure or in another way would not be eligible. This links back to nurses' issues as women. As nurses interviewed attested to and research demonstrates, African women are often unable to demand safe sex from partners, and rape is very common in South Africa. Women carry the burden of knowing that they face little control over their exposure to HIV. And nurses, who are educated on HIV transmission, know that they may be at high risk of infection, and this in turn impacts whether or not they will agree to be tested. The importance of these issues cannot be overstated. Nurses' lack of control over occupational and sexual exposure to HIV, and lack of affordable treatment, pose huge challenges to policy aimed to protect the health of these caregivers at work.

THREE PROVINCIAL HOSPITALS IN KwaZulu-Natal

> The biggest challenge is the terrible overload and strain on finances. While I don't think anywhere in the world is there ever enough money to do everything we have to do, but it seems that we have to achieve the impossible with the amount of money that we are given. (West, Manager, District Hospital)

Hospitals can be understood in terms of the economy of the communities where they are located, which in turn determines many health indicators. KZN has the highest level of inequality in the distribution of wealth and income of all of South Africa's nine provinces. In 1996 the Gini coefficient[2] for KZN was .60; in 2001 it was .63, indicating that inequalities increased during this period (KZN, 2003). South Africa is known for having among the world's greatest disparities,

---

[2] The Gini coefficient is a measure of inequality developed by the Italian statistician Corrado Gini and published in his 1912 paper "Variabilità e mutabilità." It is usually used to measure income inequality, but can be used to measure any form of uneven distribution. The Gini coefficient is a number between 0 and 1, where 0 corresponds with perfect equality (where everyone has the same income) and 1 corresponds with perfect inequality (where one person has all the income, and everyone else has zero income).

and KZN ranks worse that the average of the countries nine provinces. The Human Development Index (HDI) for KZN[3] is .57; this means it ranks below the score of the country overall (UNDP, 2004).

In 1996, 45.4% of those in KZN were classified as living in poverty;[4] in 2001 this number had grown to 49.9%. The figures for South Africa are 40.5% in 1996, and 48.9 in 2001. Further, KZN had the largest poverty gap in 1996 and was second in 2001.[5] Unemployment in KZN was 46.7% in 2002. In 1996, 93.7% of black South Africans were unemployed, and this grew to 94% in 2001. In 2001, 55% of the unemployed were women, up from 54.3 in 1996 (KZN, 2003).

Key public health statistics show that more people in KZN rely on public health than the national average, and many lack access to basic sanitary services (Cullinan, 2004). In 2001, 88% of KZN's 9.4 million people depended on provincial health care, and the provincial unemployment rate was reported at 46.7% (Ntuli, 2001). Among this population, 47% lived in rural areas, only 53.2% had access to electricity, 34.6% had piped water, and 12.7% had no toilet. The tuberculosis cure rate in 2000 was reported as only 48.8%, the lowest in the country. At the same time, HIV prevalence reported from antenatal clinics was the highest in the country (36.5%). In terms of health care workers to address these problems, the provincial averages were one public sector doctor per 4,362 people and one professional nurse per 901 people (HST, 2009). Cullinan (2004) also reports a KZN provincial budget decrease for 2003–2004.

Public health programs in KZN suffer from high dropout rates. Its TB cure rate, 49%, is the lowest in the country and the low rate is largely attributable to drop out. Large numbers of women reportedly drop out of the PMTCT program at every stage.[6] Despite having the highest antenatal HIV prevalence, only 34,000 women have completed PMTCT since the program was launched in June 2001. KZN has the greatest number of people with HIV, around 1.8 million, of whom an estimated 450,000 need antiretroviral (ARV) drugs (Cullinan, 2004).

Hospitals can also be understood historically by the shifts in political and social conditions and the health policies that these conditions and responses to them produced. Current health policy in South Africa replaced decades of colonial and apartheid policy. Colonial health policy aimed at stemming infectious disease spread and maintaining a basic level of workforce health (Gish, 2004).

---

[3] See Chapter 3 for a more complete discussion of the HDI in South Africa and international comparisons.

[4] Defined as households that expend less than R352.53 per month per adult equivalent (KZN, 2003).

[5] The poverty gap measures the distance between income and the poverty line. This indicates that KZN's poor are among the poorest in the entire country.

[6] This program relies on counseling women who are then tested for HIV, then finally agree to a single dose of niviripine for PMTCT.

Apartheid-era health policy was more explicit in maintaining race segregation in patients and staff (Marks, 1994). Beginning in the 1970s, the apartheid government sought to adapt to changing economic and social conditions brought on by increasing African militancy by creating self-ruled, ethnically defined Bantu homelands. These artificially imposed homelands were the "linchpin of apartheid social engineering in the 1960s–1970s" (Marks, 1994, p. 183). Separate departments of health were created in each of the Bantustans, part of an effort to force homeland governments to accept independence from South Africa piece by piece, and diffuse the movement for South African liberation. Nurses were an important link in the attempt to establish acceptance of the homelands by Africans. Medical sociologists have noted that educated women in the Bantustans, teachers or nurses, were a target for building alliances to the homelands as "the existence of separate health services (could) only help consolidate ethnic rather than south African loyalties" (Marks, 1994, p. 184). The result further consolidated divisions between privileged urban whites and neglected rural blacks.

Another characteristic of the South African health system and health policy is the development of one of the most sophisticated private health systems in the world. As in the United States, publicly funded medical training and research supports a highly privatized, technically advanced medical system that is at the forefront of medical science (Benatar, 2004). For example, in 1967 the first heart transplant was performed at Groote Schuur Hospital in Cape Town. Historically, the public health system has competed with the private system. Nursing shortages in South Africa dating back to the 1950s were attributed to the fact that white nurses were siphoned from the public system to the private, where pay was one third higher (Marks, 1994). Today, private-sector employment for physicians and nurses is disproportionate to the number of patients seen. Sixty-six percent of physicians work in the private sector, where only 20% receive care. Nurse/patient ratios are 1:247 overall, but 1:910 in the public sector alone (RSA, 2003b; South African Nursing Council, 2003). Of the 9% of GDP spent on health, 60% goes to the 18% who have private insurance[7] (Benatar, 2004).

South Africa has also been at the forefront of progressive public health developments. The work of Emily and Sidney Kark at Pholea, the first South African community health center created in the 1940s, to address the health needs of the disposed in their social context, contributed to the worldwide movement for primary health care (Susser, 1999). During the apartheid years, health practitioners/activists organized to address health needs in political context. South

---

[7]The degree of privatization in the South African hospital is beyond anything I have encountered. As a surgery patient in a private hospital in Durban, I observed that each service (ultrasound, phlebotomy, food service, pharmacy) was owned by a separate corporation. Without Medical Aide, many required payment at the time of service to a separate cashier. Billing was the same. The "hospital" was more or less a building housing different companies.

African policy analysts have noted that health policy had a "leg up" over other social policy areas at the time of transition to democracy due to the rich legacy of policy development and organizing by progressive public health practitioners (Stack & Hlela, 2002). The 1995 White Paper on Health Sector Transformation, the postapartheid government's guiding document for health-sector transformation, laid out principles for change aimed at increasing quality and access to health services through a district-based primary health care system with specific avenues for community involvement. There has been progress toward the goals laid out in the White Paper, notably establishing free care for mothers and children under six, and access to abortion services in the public sector. At the same time, there have been setbacks and failures in implementation that have generally been attributed to finance constraints and the demands of the HIV/AIDS epidemic.

The provincial system in KZN combined existing hospitals in the KwaZulu homeland and Natal districts into one system. In addition, new clinics were established to extend the reach of primary level services. After 1996, 145 new or replacement clinics were built (RSA, 2004). One of the primary issues for health in KZN is HIV/AIDS among poor people who until recently had no access to medication. Health services face enormous burdens due to HIV/AIDS (Bateman, 2001; Cullinan, 2004). Since 2003, funding has been made available to the provinces specifically for HIV/AIDS through a conditional grant.[8]

The resource disparities between homeland, township, and South African health services left a legacy of urban/rural inequities that carried over into the current system after existing hospitals and clinics were combined after 1994 (Stack & Hlela, 2002). During the apartheid era, disparities served as the basis for political organizing. For example, in September 1990 black nurses went on strike over discrepancies between Natal and KwaZulu salary levels (Marks, 1994, p. 204).

THE DISTRICT, REGIONAL, AND CENTRAL STUDY HOSPITALS

Three provincial hospitals were chosen for this study to generally reflect the range of differences between hospitals in the KZN public system. Table 1 shows the dimensions of difference that were considered. Hospitals were also chosen under time and resource constraints that required them to be within a reasonable driving distance of one another.

The District Hospital (DH)

DH is a 128-bed district hospital located northwest of Durban, KZN. Built by Norwegian Lutheran Missionaries in the late-19th century, DH is located near a rural village in an area cut off from the nearby coast by lush hills and sugar cane fields. In 1978 DH was taken over by the KwaZulu homeland authority.

---

[8] In 2004 conditional grants from the national government accounted for 52% of spending on AIDS at the provincial level (Idasa, 2004).

Table 1. Provincial Hospitals

Hospitals	Location	History	Function
DH (District Hospital)	Rural	Missionary (pre-1978), KwaZulu homeland (1978-1994)	District level 1 (primary level)
RH (Regional Hospital)	Small town	Natal district	Regional
CH (Central Hospital)	Urban	Built and commissioned in postapartheid era, managed as a public/private partnership	Central

Following the end of apartheid and the transition to democracy in 1994, DH joined the provincial hospital system as a Level 1 District hospital.

Beginning in 2000 the area immediately surrounding DH suffered an outbreak of cholera after a system of cost recovery for clean water taps was implemented, and many who could not afford the rates resorted to using river water (Jeter, 2002).[9] In 1999 local authorities in the area began privatization of basic services at the municipal level and signed contracts with multinational corporations including France-based Saur International and British-based Biwater (Bond, 2004b). Shortly thereafter, the surrounding area suffered a cholera outbreak: between 2000 and 2002 there were 114,000 cases, more than five times the number of cholera cases for the previous 20 years combined (see Figure 1).

At the time of my visit to DH, there was another mini-outbreak of cholera.

DH is a compound of one-story buildings and trailers that sit atop a hill. The wards at DH are small and crowded. The hospital manager describes her impression of the hospital when she first arrived to take her post:

> As I drove in, I thought, "what am I going into?" It looked like a neglected army barracks. (Ndebele, Hospital Manager)

Beyond the physical appearance, this manager, a veteran of community-based services in KZN, was also surprised by neglect of hospital issues and patient needs (see Figure 2).

---

[9]The availability of sewage systems lagged behind clean water. David Sanders, professor of public health at the University of the Western Cape explains, "People didn't have sanitation and so they shit in the river. People didn't have money to pay for their water, and so they went to the river for water" (Jeter, 2002, p. 5). At the same time, the health department response was rapid and effective, and the death toll from the outbreak was remarkably low given the numbers affected: only 260 deaths from 114,000 cases.

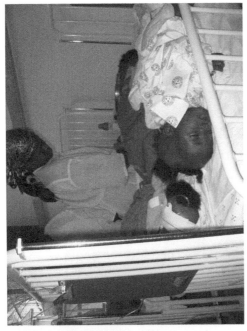

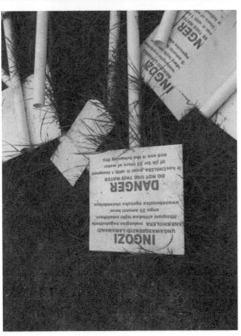

Figure 1. Photographs from the District Hospital.
Signs, lying in a pile unused at DH, with warnings not to use river water in English and Zulu and babies three to a cot. Photographs taken by the author.

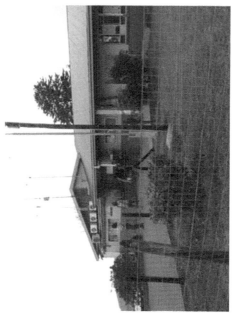
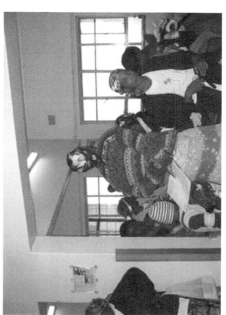

Figure 2. DH outpatient area from inside and outside. Photographs taken by the author.

When I came here, I discovered a number of things that had not been happening in the hospital. Where I came from, the community section, we always had some movement, things happening. But here there were many problems that had been neglected by the head of hospitals and local management. (Ndebele, HM)

The Regional Hospital (RH)

RH is a regional hospital located a stone's throw from the Indian Ocean along the hibiscus coast of KZN, south of Durban (see Figure 3). Located near the center of a small city that is surrounded by vacation homes on the coast and rural settlements to the west, RH is a multistoried, elevator building surrounded by one-story buildings that house casualty, AIDS clinic, nurse education, and social work. Plans for an addition to the facility have been drawn up and modeled, and are on display in the wood-lined hospital conference room. The wards, while not large, were basically comfortable and modern. Upon walk-through, the maternity and outpatient areas appeared to be overcrowded and the staff stretched thin.

Prior to the unification of KwaZulu and Natal province that formed KZN, RH was a Natal district hospital that primarily served whites. At the time of my visit, RH was recently upgraded from a district to regional hospital and was not yet fully staffed to provide the full range of regional services. RH was also preparing to join a pilot project to look at implementation of policy that requires government employees to obtain hospital services at provincial (not higher-priced private) hospitals. Private providers in the area admit to RH for medial and surgical services; and this provides an additional source of patients and fees to the hospital.

The Central Hospital

CH is a central hospital offering tertiary, quaternary, and teaching services to a region that spans KZN and half of the Eastern Cape province. CH is located just outside of Durban, the largest city in KZN, situated on the Indian Ocean. CH was planned in the apartheid era and built by the ANC-led government in 1998. The hospital began to provide service in 2002, one department at a time. The process of opening new departments is termed "commissioning," and as new services are commissioned at CH, they are decommissioned at other area tertiary facilities, shifting referrals, resources, and sometimes staff. CH is a private/public partnership (PPP) in which the province contracts out "noncore" (nonmedical) services. The hospital is entirely computerized (paperless)—including ordering systems, patient records, and films—and the management structure reflects the influence of the private sector model; the "hospital manager" at other provincial facilities is a chief executive officer (CEO) at CH. CH was built because the area lacked a central hospital for specialized referrals in the public system. However justified, dedicating resources to specialized care contradicts explicit

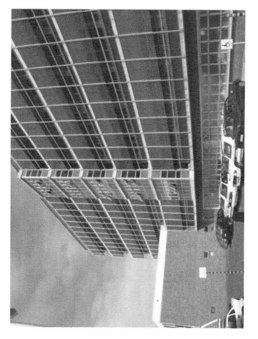

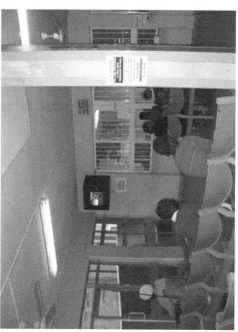

Figure 3. RH outpatient waiting area and front view of hospital. Photographs taken by the author.

commitments to the priorities of the national and provincial health policy to primary, district-based care that were spelled out in the main document on health transformation.

The words of then-vice president Jacob Zuma at the hospital dedication in 2000 are characteristic of how the hospital is regarded in South Africa (ANC, 2002):

> We are indeed extremely proud to be opening one of the most technologically sophisticated medical facilities in the world, in our country.
>
> We are gathered here from all corners of the country because we are aware of the importance of this institution to our health care system, and indeed our social development goals as a country.
>
> This paperless hospital will not only save government millions of rands, but will make a huge difference in the provision of health care in this province. (p. 2)

Physically, CH is an impressive site. It is composed of two 4-story buildings, one for administration and the other for medical services. It is an attractive, modern site, whose public function is reflected in its designed use of open space (see Figure 4).

HOSPITAL MANAGEMENT

The bulk of the information in the first two sections of this case study was provided by managers, who also play a role in defining nurses' work environment. Understanding who these people are helps to place their comments in context. All but one of the managers was South African, and between them they had a wealth of managerial and care experience. Of the managers interviewed, 10 out of 18 were nurses, a number with primary care and maternity training and experience.

Race and gender differences between the three hospitals for the same positions are apparent. The staff at DH district hospital in the management positions surveyed is overwhelmingly female and African. With the exceptions of two Cuban doctors, a white female physical therapist, and two Indian pharmacists, the entire staff was African at the time of my visit. By comparison, at RH, the staff was more white and female, and at CH the staff was more male, though only one of the men was white (see Table 2).

The racial composition of South Africa is 79% African; 9.6% white; 8.9% colored; and 2.5% Indian/Asian, based on the 2001 census (SSA, 2001). Like the rest of South Africa, the vast majority of the population of KZN is African (8,002,407 [85%]). For the remaining 15%, 8% (798,275) are Indian, 2% (141,887) are colored and 5% (483,448) are white. Over half of the population live in rural areas (5,554,0271 [56.9%]) (SSA, 2004). The racial composition of

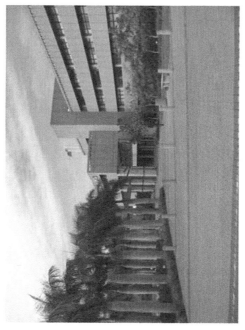

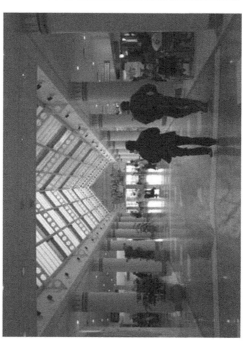

Figure 4. CH outpatient waiting area and front view of hospital. Photographs taken by the author.

Table 2. Management Demographics and Prior Experience

Name	Institution	Title	Gender	Race	Previous experience
Ndebele	DH	Hospital manager (HM)	F	A	Primary Care Nurse and administration with DoH
Megeba	DH	Nurse, H&S Committee chair (OHS)	F	A	Nurse
Sizani	DH	Nurse Manager (NM)	F	A	Nurse, Matron
Ntsele	DH	Finance Manager (FM)	M	A	Finance at hospitals with DoH
Dlamini	DH	Social Worker (SW)	F	A	First job
West	RH	Hospital Manager (HM)	F	W	Primary Care Nurse and administration with DoH
Ngubane	RH	Nurse Manager (NM)	F	A	Primary Care Nurse and administration with DoH
White	RH	Infection Control Nurse (ICH)	F	W	Private sector occupational health services, HIV/AIDS laboratory
Mitchell	RH	Finance Manager (FM)	F	W	Administration at RH
Mapley	RH	Human Resources Manager (HR)	F	W Afrikaans	Nursing Assistant, Clerk at RH
Bezuidenhout	RH	Occupational Health Services (OHS)	F	W Afrikaans	Nurse, Matron, decontamination
Holt	RH	Physician (MD)	F	W Irish	MD with DoH, hospital, researcher
Robinson	CH	Chief Executive Officer (CEO)	M	British	British NHS
Zuma	CH	Occupational Health Services (OHS)	F	A	Private sector occupational health services
Mazibuko	CH	Nurse Manager (NM)	F	A	Nurse with DoH
Ndlovu	CH	Infection Control Nurse (ICN)	F	A	Infection control nurse, Guateng
Singh	CH	Human Resources (HR)	M	I	Provincial department of transport, forestry
Radebe	CH	Finance Manager (FM)	M	A	Finance manager at other hospitals with DoH
Clark	CH	Private Partner (PP)	M	W	Private sector

the management positions at these three hospitals reflect the surrounding areas in expected ways. However, the differences between the three hospitals are illustrative of the environments of each. The district hospital remains African in patient and management profile. The regional hospital carries the burden of a race-segregated hierarchy, though the additions of female and African female hospital managers and nurse managers are a conscious departure from the past. The central hospital better reflects the racial composition of South Africa, though women were less well-represented than they were in the other two hospitals.

Comparison of the backgrounds of hospital managers reveals a wealth of experience in the public system. Additionally, the hospital managers at both the district and regional hospitals were experienced primary-care nurses, as was the nurse manager at the central hospital.

Race, gender, and experience of management are important in assessing their comments about nurses, patients, and hospital challenges. It is fair to say that management, particularly at the regional and district level hospitals, had an understanding of nurse and medical issues that was steeped in medical experience and cultural understanding. At the same time, management positions and age differences had a bearing on their views. Nurse managers at RH and DH were critical of the commitment of younger nurses to patient care and the nursing profession. The hospital manager at RH (who also has training in social science) traced the deterioration of nurses' commitment to the involvement of African nurses in strikes during 1980s. Though these comments express generational and labor/management conflict, they also express sympathy and comradery. They also provide insight into the totality of hospital nurses historical experiences.

> When I was trained we were almost brainwashed into ethical standards about what should be done, what shouldn't be done, and our responsibility to the patient. It was really almost a calling rather than a job . . . . You can never generalize; of course there were horrible nurses when I trained, but generally the more mature nurses seem to be more dedicated, more ethical, and are willing to put up with more stress and hard work than younger nurses.
>
> When we were really politically hot, before democratization, the only political power that African people had was through the trade unions. It was pretty violent, and nurses were not initially pressurized to join the strikes. Nurses didn't want to join the strikes because we believed that we were endangering the lives of people. But also, the comrades were of the belief that the nurses needed to be there, in the hospital, when they were injured. But over the years that went away and there was more and more pressure on nurses to strike. Some did so, really reluctantly, but once you've done it, it becomes easier and easier. As the years went on, nurses did really easily go on strike, literally walking out of nurseries, leaving no one to care for babies, and babies did die. People did die as a result.
>
> However legitimate that may have been for the country, it definitely changed the mind of the profession. We lost something as a profession. I honestly believe that there is less commitment to the welfare of the patient.

Things are happening that never would have happened prior to that kind of transformation unionization. It's not the unionization, it's the political pressure. Some nurses who refused to strike had threats against their lives and their families. Terrible pressure was put on them. The great body of the profession changed. The mindset changes, and neglect became common.[10] (West, HM)

Health Care Challenges

Despite the considerable differences between the three hospitals in this study, key management personnel at each described providing quality care in the context of inadequate government support and a serious shortage of nurses as the main challenge faced at their respective institutions.[11] However, these challenges were characterized in ways that were significantly different in each setting. These differences reflect varying degrees of institutional-level problems with staff shortages, finances, and head office responsiveness. In the case of DH, differences are underscored by a severely and relatively deprived environment.

At DH, managers described how scarce resources and lack of space impacted patient care, including an actual decline in medical services from previous periods:

We have an issue with quality that relates to space. We have many new programs—occupational therapist, dietician—and they only have little corners. How do we do this? When I came there wasn't even a screen between the beds, so this is one of the first things we attended to. Even in a small area, we have to give some privacy. Another issue linked to quality is the shortage of personnel from all angles. Not the administrative side, that is easy. But from the professional side, there is a shortage of doctors, and nurses of all categories. This is linked to quality, because if you are trying to stretch the few people that you have, you get burn-out, and then they leave. So you need to stretch them to a reasonable state. (Ndebele, HM)

We don't have most of the equipment. We are short of skilled personnel, especially doctors. Because of this we cannot perform some of the procedures. We cannot do surgery because we don't have a surgeon. We don't have an obstetrician, we do only minor things, we can't do a c-section. We have no anesthesiologist. Even relocations we can't do. We did all these things before. Things have gotten worse, generally because of staff shortages. (Sizani, NM)

[10] This statement is interesting in its similarities to statements from nurse managers in the United States who decry the impact of unions on nursing practice. At the same time, the analysis in relation to South Africa's political turmoil is different. I don't think these views can be put down simply to a labor vs. management perspective, though full analysis is beyond the purpose here. It is clear that this empathetic observer notes that commitment of nurses has suffered in postapartheid South Africa, that there were costs to the transformation process.

[11] This was in direct response to the question, "What is the greatest challenge you face in your job?"

Mrs. Ndebele, the hospital manager, rooted these concerns in lack of support for the hospital that she attributed to the National Department of Health's lack of support to the province.

> The biggest challenge is that the institution would like to see some support coming from head office. We have a problem when it comes to support, which is that workers will be looking at local management and saying we aren't giving support, and local managers are looking at head office, province to national. (Ndebele, HM)

Lack of support for the hospital was expressed in interviews by the phrase "nothing is happening," used by both the hospital manager and nurse manager. Mrs. Ndebele, the hospital manager, described how a mini-outbreak of cholera was exacerbating the lack of space at the hospital. Despite the fact that three children share a cot in the pediatric ward and that she had contacted the provincial health department about the serious medical risk of cross infection, she explained,

> Nothing is happening; last we heard, a contractor would arrive later this year, but nothing is happening. I understand that we aren't the only hospital with a space problem, so I suppose we need to prioritize. I understand at head office they are being pushed from all angles, but when you are sitting on the ground you really feel that you are not being supported. (Ndebele, HM)

The DH nurse manager's description of changes at the hospital over her 36-year tenure underscores the hospital manager's assessment of neglect and lack of support.

> Not much has changed. When I came it was a Norwegian Lutheran hospital. Then there was a laundry built, it was built by the government in 1978, because we had a very poor laundry in which we had pots, we used to boil our linen, they were hand-washed. So we were just doing that, boiling, washing, rinsing, hanging outside. No machinery, nothing. So after the take-over of the government in 1978, nothing happened; but early in the 1980s they built that laundry for us. (Sizani, NM)

When asked what had changed since the government transition in 1994, Mrs. Sizani indicated that nothing distinguished this period from the period of homeland management under apartheid:

> So far nothing. Except for those park homes that are used as offices, and these others that are used as residences, and that small house for the doctors. Otherwise, nothing. (Sizani, NM)

These comments are striking given the tumultuous political and social events of this period, and the expectation that the end of apartheid would result in attention to disadvantaged rural Africans.

One issue that was not raised in the interviews that may have bearing on provincial support/neglect of DH was local politics. Political power within the KZN provincial government is shared between the Inkatha Freedom Party (IFP)[12] and the ANC. This division has ethnic and geographical distinctions; IFP had historically been the party of the Zulu people in KZN, ANC of the Xhosa people, concentrated in the Eastern Cape as well as other apartheid foes of all backgrounds. Some reports about DH suggest that this hospital has been neglected within local political structures because of ANC leadership through the DoH, and its location in a mainly IFP region (*Daily News*, 2000).

At RH, managers echoed the DH manager's opinion that providing quality patient care amidst scarce resources of staff and finance was a great challenge.

> The biggest challenge is the terrible overload and strain on finances. While I don't think anywhere in the world is there ever enough money to do everything we have to do, but it seems that we have to achieve the impossible with the amount of money that we are given. I think you can see that we have squeezed up every bit of accommodation that we can. Our outpatient department is completely underresourced for the amount of patients that we have to deal with. Our maternity unit is completely underresourced and too small. We have a serious problem with recruitment of professional nurses. It's trying to provide a reasonable quality of care when you don't have the personnel to provide it. (West, HM)

However, far from occurring in a context where "nothing is happening," at RH the hospital is upgrading from district to regional status, participating in a pilot project to introduce a new requirement that government employees use provincial hospitals for medical services and admit private patients from the community. In short, the insufficiency of resources is related to expansion, change, and response to increased need.

The hospital manager and finance manager expressed uncertainty over the resource support that RH would receive from the province during its transition phase.

> Our next biggest challenge is turning the hospital around from a community to regional hospital. . . . We were led to believe that we would have suffi-cient resources last year, since they roughly give you an idea of what you

[12] The IFP, led by Mangosuthu Gatsha Buthelezi from 1970 to 1994, served as the chief leader for the KwaZulu homeland or Bantustan. The IFP was a Zulu nationalist organization that favored a tribal solution to apartheid. The IFP opposed the ANC and was accused of collaboration with white supremacists, and was involved in violent clashes during the transition period. These differences were appeased, and Buthelezi served in the postapartheid government as home affairs minister through Mbeki's first term. KZN is currently split politically between the ANC and IFP in a coalition government, and politics is very contentious and generally related to ethnic background.

> will have. That would have been sufficient for us in a very meaningful way
> to start transforming. But as we get nearer and nearer to the new year, the
> amount of money has shrunk to the point where we have no more than last
> year. Verbally we have been told that as we establish regional services, we
> can create business plans and try to compete for additional funds. In theory,
> those funds should come from the Durban complex because we will be
> sending them less work, but I think that is in theory. (West, HM)

> We have had no changes for increasing needs. Even with salary changes,
> we work on a fixed budget. They ask you to give an estimate. We give them
> one, but it doesn't come near. We work over-budget now, especially with
> medicines. We overspend all the time. Even with vacant posts, we are
> overspending. There is always an increase in July. Now, already in May,
> we are short. (Mitchell, FM)

At CH, commissioning a new hospital in the context of a nursing shortage
and an insufficient budget was described as the greatest challenge facing the
institution. However, lack of space and patient overload were not issues at CH.
Although the hospital is aiming at 85% average occupancy, it was operating at
below 50% at the time of this study in 2003, with some empty beds accounted for
by departments not yet transferred from former locations (Singh, HR). Based
on observation, only the outpatient area appeared busy, and the wards and units
had many empty beds.

Another difference between CH and its provincial counterparts in this study
was the sense of head office responsiveness. This quote from the finance manager,
Mr. Radebe, suggests that the provincial and national offices are aware of
budgetary problems and inclined to respond to CH needs.

> We don't have the budget for the number of staff that are needed. There is also
> a general consensus that salaries are not adequate to retain staff. This is why
> nurses are leaving abroad, but this is a separate issue. For us, the main problem
> is that the money we have and the number of staff do not match. This can only
> be resolved by a reduction in staff and services, or national action to correct
> the conditional grant. We have brought this to the province's attention, and
> national has agreed that grants of the largest provinces should be reviewed.
> (Radebe, FM)

Over 6 days of observation of CH, the Superintendent General's car was
observed on multiple days, providing further evidence that a different level of
responsiveness existed at the central hospital: the highest ranking DoH official
was directly available to CH management. In a U.S. appearance at Harvard Law
School, Minister of Finance Trevor Manuel touted the successful public/private
partnership (PPP) at CH as evidence of the country's progress in economic
development. Business journals in South Africa ran favorable reports on the
CH model of PPP; CH is typically mentioned in a list of South African PPPs
that also includes highways (N3 toll road), prisons (Louis Trichardt APOPS

Prison), and water (Dolphin Coast Water Concession) (*Business Day*, 2004). The newness, complex issues involved with commissioning high-level medical and teaching services, technology, and high stakes/high profile investment in the PPP model and world-class facility provide further reasons for greater head office responsiveness at CH than at other KZN provincial hospitals.

Finances

Financial resources are a reflection of economic policy in the health system, thus they are given special consideration here. This policy reflects the priorities of the Department of Health. The health budget in KZN in 2003 was inadequate to fund provincial hospitals; they were overbudget, and this shortfall was predicted to persist and increase (KZN, 2003). In part this was due to increased usage based on HIV/AIDS. It was also due to the fact that the central hospital was behind schedule opening, so tertiary services were duplicated.

Budgets

District and regional hospitals operate from a budget determined by their size (number of beds) and service level (Stack & Hlela, 2002). Their funding comes from a provincial allocation through a global budget from the national government; the health sector competes with other sectors for these funds, and hospitals compete against other health services within the provincial budget. At the national level, the amount of the global budget to the provinces is affected by other demands and constraints on the national budget, such as debt repayment and policies intended to curb inflation (Poggenpoel & Claasen, 2004). The central hospital, like all others in South Africa, operates under a conditional grant from the national department of health that is separate from the provincial budget. There is also a conditional grant specifically for HIV/AIDS. The yearly budget of the 128-bed DH is R30 million; for the 229-bed RH, it is R82 million; and for the 846-bed CH, it is R300 million (Cullinan, 2004; KZN, 2003; Mitchell, FM; Radebe, FM).

At RH and CH, finance and hospital managers reported operating with budgets that were inadequate for the type and volume of services they provided. At CH, management appeared to have more faith in their ability to obtain budget increases from national-level grants than RH did from provincial-level grants

Income

All hospitals charge for services based on a fee scale that considers income and medical-aid coverage. Fees are collected by the hospitals and are sent to the Provincial Department of Health, and they are intended to offset the costs of providing services. Even DH, a district hospital serving a poor rural population, reported taking in R13,000 to R14,000 in fees per month (Ntsele, FM).

Medical Aide presents the potential for additional revenue to the public system, though in this case, provincial hospitals compete with private hospitals (RSA, 2004). Though far more expensive,[13] the private health care system is generally a more attractive environment, which employs far more physicians and has a competitive advantage (Benatar, 2004). Still, some provincial hospitals are able to compete in specific ways. For example, managers at RH described how private physicians frequently admit their patients to RH for care at the facility; CH, with its attractive new facility, specialized services, and relationship with the Nelson Mandela School of Medicine—specifically academic doctors—has features that enhance its competitiveness with the private sector. The lower costs of provincial services compared with private-hospital services present an opportunity for profit by HMO-style insurance; a recent National DoH document references how this relates to new medical schemes regulation (RSA, 2004):

> A major thrust of medical schemes legislation has been to ensure that schemes do not discriminate among members and that they provide an essential package of benefits to all members. The minimum benefit provision has prompted medical schemes to seek health care providers that offer the best value for money and designate them as preferred providers. (p. 64)

Thus, the document notes new "engagement between the public and private sectors" in health care. Currently the province is introducing this type of arrangement through the Medical Aide offered to government employees. In the future, government employees may have to use provincial hospital facilities for care (Mitchell FM). This presents an opportunity for the Medical Aide to save on hospital costs, and for the government to recoup some of the two thirds proportion it pays for employee health benefits. At the same time, since labor is the largest cost in the health care service budget, it stands to follow that cheaper labor is an important factor in the lower cost of provincial health services. Thus, successful competition depends on lower wages to public health care workers.

IMPACTS OF HIV/AIDS ON THE THREE HOSPITALS

Impacts of HIV/AIDS on Hospital Services

The increases in number of patients with HIV/AIDS in KZN provincial hospitals has caused a drain of resources available for other ailments, rise in costs due to lengthy stays, and expensive medications for opportunistic infections and other care. It has worsened working conditions for the staff, and altered the hospital work environment.

---

[13] For example, a cesarean delivery costs R16,000 in the private sector, R3,500 in the public (Mitchell, FM).

HIV/AIDS effects the hospitals differently because of the level of services offered. At the district and regional hospital, HIV/AIDS patients are admitted for opportunistic infections related to HIV and advanced AIDS. These patients are typically very sick and require palliative care (McNeill, 2002). At the central hospital, fewer AIDS patients are seen because the hospital operates on referrals for specialty care (Mazibuko, NM). Exceptions are the outpatient clinics at CH, where patients cannot be turned away. Patients use the clinics as primary services despite the fact that it is discouraged. The other exception is the neonatal intensive care (NICU), where HIV+ newborns are attended to and where mothers are tested for HIV, and PMTCT is administered.[14]

Hospital managers at the district and regional hospitals in this study described how HIV/AIDS and the opportunistic infections it engenders had intensified care and worsened working conditions for staff. Public hospitals in South Africa face a significant burden from the HIV/AIDS epidemic; studies in KZN have shown that AIDS is the most common reason for admission (Floyd, Reid, Wilkinson, & Gilks, 1999), which have risen dramatically with the explosion of the HIV/AIDS epidemic (Colvin, Dawood, Kleinschmidt, Mullick, & Lallo, 2001).

At DH and RH, management described how patients were sicker and stayed in the hospital longer. The resultant financial burdens and discharge of terminally ill patients were described as attendant issues by hospital managers.

> The severity of the illness has had a huge impact on our hospital. AIDS patients are severely, severely ill. The drugs they require are more costly than many other patients, so it has financial implications. They take longer to recover, so the length of stay is longer. If they are in the end stages—we have a large population of terminally ill patients—we need not to be treating them, because this is an acute-care hospital. But these patients come from such terrible financial circumstances that there is nowhere to discharge to; it would be inhumane. (West, HM)

In KZN, as in much of South Africa, AIDS/TB is a significant problem. It is estimated that TB incidence has approximately tripled in KZN over the past 8 years (Fourie & Weyer, 2002). This increase is consistent with scientific modeling, which shows an HIV prevalence of 20% leading to more than doubling of the average size of TB outbreaks (Porco, 2001). Tuberculosis is the most common illness that signals the onset of AIDS in KZN and in all of sub-Saharan Africa. Since AIDS prevalence lags HIV prevalence by 3 to7 years, even if the HIV prevalence stabilizes in the province, the AIDS/TB epidemic will not peak until 2004–2010 (O'Donnell & Zelnick, 2002). The major factors that contribute to HIV-associated TB include the fact that latent TB is up to 200 times more likely to become active TB with HIV co-infection (Corbett, Steketee, Ter Kuile,

---

[14] A single dose of the ARV neviripine is given to the mother and baby in order to reduce transmission of HIV during childbirth.

Latif, Kamali, & Hayes, 2002); the high risk of rapidly progressive TB in HIV+ patients; high recurrence rates, and higher transmission rates of TB in the hospital and community.

At DH, management indicated that they had found 90% of TB patients are HIV+.

> Because of HIV/AIDS, and our patients are sicker for a longer period, it is difficult to know for the medical side because every patient is not tested for HIV. But for the TB side, 90% are HIV positive. We have a VCT site, and we counsel them as they come in. Most of them get tested, but not routinely, only with permission. But because we have counselors here and a TB team, we are able to get a number of them. We have a dedicated TB ward, and most of our patients there are HIV positive, and they occupy the space for longer periods, though we would like them out as quickly as possible. (Ndebele, HM)

Outbreaks of cholera were referenced at both the district hospital and the regional hospital that also serves a rural, poor population. At DH, a small cholera outbreak occurred at the time of this study and exacerbated other problems faced by the hospital.

> We now are having a mini-outbreak of cholera, and the children are coming in very quickly. The small children are sleeping three in a bed, there will be cross-infection. Any mother can stay at the hospital if she is breastfeeding, otherwise others must go home. So now what we see is that all the mothers are breastfeeding. But I went in there to say, "But guys, if you are all breastfeeding, how do the children have cholera?" (Ndebele, HM)

> We are still seeing a lot of diarrhea, even without cholera. Basically it is linked to the development out in the community. (Ndebele, HM)

Impacts of HIV/AIDS on Hospital Staff

The increase in HIV/AIDS in provincial hospitals changed the work performed by nurses and other health care staff. Hospital managers at DH and RH described the stressful working conditions created by the HIV/AIDS epidemic. The hospital manager at RH noted the triple threat imposed by HIV/AIDS on patients, family members, and themselves.

> From a morale point of view, it depresses the doctors and nurses. The hopelessness and dealing with all these terminally ill patients all the time really has an impact on them. Added to that, most nursing staff are African. Very many themselves are affected by the virus. Infected and affected. Their families, always close family members are dying, there are orphans involved. (West, HM)

The phrase "infected and affected" was used on multiple occasions by a number of managers. Managers described how nurses worked with AIDS patients all week, and took time off to attend funerals on the weekend. In addition to the burdens of increased patient numbers and acuity, nurse manager Mrs. Sizani described the difficulties of nursing HIV+ patients who do not want to know their HIV status.

> HIV/AIDS had added more pressure on our personnel, because they work under stressful conditions now. We have to cater for HIV/AIDS patients as well. And they need more care and more attention because they are always very, very ill. And they usually come in with these opportunistic diseases, so we have to treat that as well. . . . Patients are still reluctant to know their HIV status, this is the toughest thing of all. Because it is easier to nurse a patient who knows. You are free to give advice and to do everything for them. Rather than say, "Oh, it is this, but I really cannot say." It is really stressful for the nurses. (Sizani, NM)

The dilemma of sick patients who refuse to be tested for HIV is a key fact in understanding HIV/AIDS care in the hospital and its impact on nurses' work environment. The stigma attached to the disease in the community also characterizes it in the hospital. The dynamics of stigmatization are complex, but are characterized by the sexual spread of the disease and women's oppressed social position (Susser, 2002). Myths related to rumor, and at times traditional medical advice,[15] compete with scientific understanding of the disease. Whatever the source of stigma, it is reinforced in practice in the hospital.

Discrimination against PLWA, ranging from discriminatory hiring practices to one documented case of a woman who was stoned to death after publicly disclosing her status (SAPA, 2001), has engendered a culture of confidentiality.[16] Confidentiality plays an important role in protecting PLWA and guaranteeing their human rights. At the same time, it also serves to reinforce an environment of secrecy and the sense that there is something wrong that must be kept private. This can be best understood in contrast to other diseases. People frequently keep their health status confidential to protect against discrimination, but the added stigma of HIV/AIDS complicates how confidentiality is understood. In an environment of secrecy and stigma, an official policy of confidentiality denotes that talking or writing about HIV status is forbidden, and clouds the issue of open discussion and the benefits it could bring.

Medical doctor Laura Holt, from RH, discussed how the issue of confidentiality had acted as a distraction in efforts to set up a palliative care team at the hospital.

---

[15] Traditional healers have a strong role in Zulu culture. Traditional healers have been successfully integrated in health campaigns in KZN, South Africa (Colvin, Gumede, Grimwade, Maher, & Wilkinson, 2003).

[16] Examples of the range of confidentiality policies are footnoted in Chapter 6.

Nurses' openness to discussing HIV/AIDS? It's not there. When we started palliative care, we suggested to put AIDS patients together, and we were told that we were stigmatizing them. Here we are, 15 years into this epidemic, these people are dying of AIDS, and you're saying that I am stigmatizing them by putting them in a cubicle so I can care for them better! . . . It's still on this secret level, where we have to write "condoms prescribed." The social worker that came, the very first question she asked was, "are we allowed to write the HIV result in our note?" We take people out of outpatient casualty to be counseled with family. To tell them, "It looks like you have AIDS, there is not much we can do." But the nurses are saying, "You can't do that, you are breaking the person's confidentiality with their family." They don't realize that this person is dying, in a wheelchair, in their last week of life . . . I think it is ignorance. People are not understanding, not seeing the depth of the problem. They are looking at insignificant things, like what do I write in the note. Meanwhile we've had to empty the mortuary twice this week—15 people have died. (Holt, MD)

While Dr. Holt was frustrated in her role, she also expressed understanding of why nurses might need to use the official confidentiality policy to protect their relationships with patients that extended to the community outside of the hospital.

HIV/AIDS has been hijacked by counselors and social workers. It isn't a medical thing. I feel frustrated that I can't help AIDS patients because I "can't do this," "not allowed to do that." How can I care for this person while their mother doesn't know? How can you care for people properly when the family doesn't know? As a doctor, it's frustrating to deal with these things. But it's totally different for a nurse. They have to go back into the community and face the same people at home. There is a lot more to it, relations and ties with people that they see in the hospital. Nurses have it more difficult than we do. (Holt, MD)

This reference to the different meanings of the epidemic to subgroups of South African health workers is an unexplored aspect of the impact of the epidemic on their work environment.

Managers also perceived that nurses did not discuss HIV/AIDS with patients, and in fact often avoided such conversations:

With community nursing, we use a WHO/UNICEF approach to treating sick children, called IMCI, Integrated Management of Childhood Illness. We've introduced questions and management related to HIV because of the huge problem of HIV in children. When you assess nurses using the approach, assessment after assessment, they avoid the HIV questions. And if you question—a researcher at our poly-technikon did research on why nurses avoided these questions—a common response was, "If I ask these questions, a mother might think her child is HIV positive," and then if you ask if this is a bad thing, they say yes, because if she thinks her child is HIV, she will think that she is HIV positive; that will upset the mother, she will be depressed, and she won't be able to take care of herself and her baby. (West, HM)

Unwilling to discuss HIV/AIDS with their patients, nurses cannot encourage them to be tested or promote open discussion of the disease. This has implications for care, the level of stress in the work environment, and nurses regard for their own health and safety.

CHAPTER 5

∝ ⁊

Staffing, Occupational Health, and HIV/AIDS

They are leaving for overseas, for Saudi Arabia, for better salaries. They lack green pastures. (Sizani, NM)

Staffing Background

South Africa has a higher density of nurses and other health workers than many countries in the region (WHO, 2003), but hospitals still face shortages in terms of the services they provide and vacancies determined by the Department of Health (Huddart & Picazo, 2003). According to the South African Nursing Council, 177,721 nurses were registered in 2003. Between 1998 and 2003 the Council's nursing registry grew by 2.3% while the South African population increased by 10.2% (42.13 million to 46.43 million) (SANC, 2004). In 2003 the Council estimated that 2,300 nurses already worked overseas, and that 200 new applications arrived per month to allow more to work abroad (UNDP, 2004).

Vacant positions are common for both nurses and physicians: of 1,258 permanent physician posts in KZN, 51.67% (650) were vacant in 2003, as were 26.91% of 11,808 "professional" nurse posts and 26.17% of 8,419 posts for "staff" and student nurse positions (KZN, 2003). Many who left were not replaced. Of 8,520 permanent professional nurses employed by the provincial department of health, 1,196 terminated or transferred out, while only 621 transferred in (KZN, 2003).

Shortages are not limited to the public sector. Private companies are offering incentives such as a 14th paycheck,[1] or 2 months work in a higher-paid overseas subsidiary (Shevel, 2003). In 2003 the private company Netcare petitioned the KZN DoH to recruit nurses from India to fill vacant positions. Meanwhile, international recruiters based in Durban (KZN's largest city) and advertisers in the

---

[1] In South Africa people commonly receive 13 monthly paychecks, the 13th is a Christmas bonus.

monthly publication of the country's combined nurse organization/union (DENOSA) make international positions easily available. In 2003 the department of health debated providing nurses with unpaid leave to work overseas so that they do not have to resign their posts (Thom, 2003).

Occupational Health and Safety Background

The earliest Occupational Health and Safety protections in South Africa were won by white craft-based trade unions and were racially exclusionary (Myers & Macun, 1989). Before the rise of the Afrikaner-led government in 1948, the context of these developments was white elite vs. white labor and the Afrikaner agrarian movement. After 1948 the context was the collusion of the state and corporations and the shrinking of the white working class. The rise of the independent black unions beginning in the late 1960s brought a spate of legislation that was aimed at taming and co-opting the new threat of black power. The economic backdrop of growth in the 1960–1970s, recession in the late 1970s, and privatization in the 1980s was important, as was the state of emergency brought about by the labor-based struggle against apartheid (Myers & Macun, 1989).

There are important consequences for current OHS policy based on history. Though the independent black labor movement has been a strong example of social unionism, was key to ushering in democracy, and plays an important role in the new government, its contributions to OHS policy have been minimal (Myers & Macun, 1993). COSATU member unions did not play a big role in developing OHS, especially since their participation was as independents, non-participants and policies that existed were developed by state or white unions. Two threats observed by occupational health progressives is that technical and socially "neutral" legislation is a barrier to more dynamic participation of non-scientists in policymaking, and that workers are excluded from OHS policy and implementation. The fact that many union leaders left for work in government, depleting the experienced, shop-floor, and province-level leadership contributes to these threats (Myers & Macun, 1993).

As has been the case worldwide, economic insecurity, unemployment, and down-sizing (retrenchment in South African language) has meant that OHS has been put on the back burner, as unions fight for survival for themselves and the working class (Qotole, 2001). While OHS committees are required in national legislation, unions are not explicitly involved. In practice, this puts additional demands on already taxed shop stewards, and means that the OHS committee reps and labor management reps are not as aligned as they might be (Henwood, 2002).

Nurse Shortages and Recruitment

The local dynamics of shortage and migration played out in a regional context, where the competitive advantages between hospitals had direct bearing on the experience of each institution in attracting and retaining staff. The labor market for nurses in KZN is characterized by overseas opportunity and heavy recruiting, especially of the most skilled staff. Each hospital in this study faced a shortage of nurses due to overseas migration. Although managers interviewed identified HIV/AIDS as a factor in nurses' working conditions, finances—specifically the quest to earn a better salary—was the unequivocal reason that managers identified for nurses seeking work abroad. Regional movement, on the other hand, was reported to be based more on differences in immediate working conditions and local quality of life, since the salaries for nurses are the same in the provincial hospitals. Finally, the opportunity to moonlight present in urban and semiurban settings, where private employers are available, offered a financial advantage for movement from a rural to an urban setting.

Table 1 provides a comparison of vacancy and attrition rates at the three hospitals in this study.

The rates of vacancy of staff positions at KZN provincial hospitals compare with an overall vacancy rate of nearly 20% for all health personnel in KZN reported in 2001 (KZN, 2002), and nursing shortages of around 27% for professional and nonprofessional categories (KZN, 2003). In the regional and district hospitals, vacancy rates were high and turnover significant despite the fact that hospital census rates either were stable or grew (Colvin et al., 2001). This indicates that the workload increased for the remaining nurses. Retired nurses who are rehired on a contract basis bring years of experience and help with the sheer number of vacancies as well as skill shortages. Managers reported shortages of nurses, especially in the professional category, that had the most skills.

Manager's indicated that budgets were not adjusted to reflect the increased HIV-related need.

Table 1. Nursing Vacancies and Attrition Rates[a]

	Hospital		
Impacts	Urban tertiary/quaternary care hospital	Small city regional hospital	Rural district hospital
Positions vacant	0/1148	25/344 (7%)	65/158 (41%)
	12.5% of nursing staff are retired nurses hired on contract basis	60% of vacancies are professional nurse category	68% of vacancies are professional nurse category
Attrition 2000-2002	20 (<2%)	112/344 (33%)	46/158 (29%)

[a]Secondary data collected from hospital managers.

Reprinted by permission from Macmillan Publishers Ltd: Jennifer Zelnick and Max O'Donnell, The Impact of the HIV/AIDS Epidemic on Hospital Nurses in KwaZulu Natal, South Africa: Nurses' Perspectives and Implications for Health Policy, *Journal of Public Health Policy, 26,* 163-185, copyright 2005. Published by Palgrave Macmillan.

> We don't have the budget for the number of staff that are needed. There is also a general consensus that salaries are not adequate to retain staff. (Radebe, FM)

> We have had no changes for increasing needs. (Mitchell, FM)

Remaining nurses must shoulder the responsibility of increased workloads due to vacant staff positions and increased need. Further, low salaries were implicated as the cause of shortages and a barrier to recruitment. Nurses are required to do more with less, with inadequate financial reward.

Hospital-Level Shortage Dynamics

Hospital nurse positions at the DH were extremely difficult to fill because nurses left for work in urban centers or overseas for quality-of-life and financial reasons. Of the three hospitals, DH had the most long-standing vacant posts.

> Enrolled nurses? Twenty-one posts are vacant; I cannot fill them. With the professional nurses it is worse, it is really worse. I am supposed to have 56: of the 56, 44 are vacant. (Sizani, NM)

Hospital managers at DH characterized how this shortage disrupted ward-level staffing.

> We are short of professional nurses, and this contributes to health and safety issues. Nurses are very overworked here. We are short-staffed, sometimes we have to nurse 20 patients while there are only 3 on the wards. Eight nurses would be the correct number for 20 patients. Nurses are stressed. (Megeba, HS)

> We must cater for night duty and day duty as well. Our services are not covered, especially the wards. Starting from maternity, we are supposed to be having a CPN, then 2 SPN, and 9 professional nurses, but they are not there. We have just one CPN and 3 professional nurses. (Sizani, NM)

It is important to note that for the numbers of staff reported on the wards, managers are referring to the full 24-hour period. The reference to 3 nurses for 20 patients refers to 24 hours, not an 8- or 12-hour shift.

The nurse manager noted that hospital nurses sometimes resigned and collected a severance package, only to reapply for entry-level positions 3 or 4 months later. This practice, not mentioned at other facilities, contributed to vacant senior posts.

> Some have resorted to resigning, going back home, then reapplying. They apply for resignation to get the severance package and the pension. But when you reapply, you lose the seniority you have accrued. (Sizani, NM)

Unlike the other hospitals in this study, DH had a significant shortage of physicians. Although 80% of patients receive care in the public hospitals, 70% of physicians work in the private sector (Benatar, 2004). One policy that offers some relief is the requirement that doctors in training contribute a "community year" to the provincial system. Another method of alleviating physician shortages is the national policy that recruits Cuban doctors to fill South African physician shortages.[2] At the time of my visit, the hospital was relying on two full-time Cuban physicians living onsite for the bulk of patient care. Other physician posts were reported vacant for 2 years.

> We are still using foreign doctors to assist us, doctor posts have been vacant for 2 years. (Ntsele, FM)

At RH, the nursing shortage was caused by increasing international migration, especially of the professional nursing categories, and the sudden loss of large numbers of nurses who came from the neighboring Eastern Cape.[3] At an extreme, the nurse manager at RH described how five nurses left in one day, though she identified a more typical figure as two per month. Both the HR and nurse manager identified 2000 as the year when nurses began to leave.

> The trend that I am seeing now is that we are getting these 24-hour notices, because someone has been processing their overseas paperwork, and suddenly she is required to leave, and it is disrupting us like anything. . . . Last month I nearly tear my hair apart, because I had 5 resignations in one day, all in one day! You are thinking, "How am I going to fill this post? What will happen to patient care?" As it is, I am sitting with 17 vacancies. And we can't recruit anywhere. . . . In fact, when it started, it was abrupt. Suddenly people were going away. But we had enough coming in from Eastern Cape so that we did not feel the impact that much. We were losing in the sense that experienced people who had been there for a long time were leaving, but we could replace them. Now we are starting to see that the well is getting dry. (Ngubane, NM)

[2] As of November 2004 there were 240 Cuban doctors working in South Africa as part of a bilateral program in which Cuban professionals are temporarily employed in South Africa through a government program. South Africa has also financed a program that has brought 100 Cuban doctors to Mali. See http://www.southafrica.info/public_services/foreigners/immigration/cuban-doctors.htm

[3] As the nurse manager explained, until recently many Eastern Cape nurses had sought work in KZN. At RH, these nurses mitigated the impacts of the nursing shortage. The NM assumed that conditions had improved in the Eastern Cape, and these nurses had been lured home. Interestingly, another recent study found that Eastern Cape nurses sought jobs in KZN because they perceived that they could more easily get in contact with international recruiters in KZN.

We are having a large turnover of nurses. There were 5 or 6 resignations per month; 53 or 54 last year. It has increased over the last 3 years. They are required to give 1 month notice, but the way it works is they wait for it to come through and book a flight, they work until the last day. (Mapley, HR)

There is a new exodus as well. I don't know what is happening in the Eastern Cape. Previously Eastern Cape nurses were coming, flocking to our services, though it was to our advantage. But all of a sudden, they are going back. Conditions have improved there, and they want to go back to their hospitals. (Ngubane, NM)

In addition to leaving for international positions, the nurse manager indicated that nurses sought work at the central hospital (also part of this study).

Many go to (the central hospital), they have nice flats that are subsidized. People like to go there, everything is nice there. Here, our accommodation is very limited—they are forced to get outside accommodation which is very expensive. (Ngubane, NM)

The urban specialty-care hospital opened in 2002 (and was slated to be fully functional in August 2003) and did not report any shortages, although not all departments were fully functional in May 2003. Although units at existing tertiary care hospitals were closed and some staff from these relocated to the new hospital, staff from other hospitals also relocated there and contributed to shortages in less desirable areas/facilities. The hospital relied on retired nurses to fill its ranks; a full 12.5% of nurses employed at the time of my 2003 visit were previously retired. Managers were aware of the potential problems for their facility, because the most highly skilled nurses have the best advantages overseas.

Nursing allows training and it is paid, so it is open to disadvantaged people. Now with the international poaching of nurses, it is that people have skilled themselves. It is skilled people, from theater (surgery), ICU, these are the ones that go. (Zuma, OHS)

In spite of advertising, we have vacant posts in professional categories—especially theaters and ICUs. That's where the shortage is felt in this country—all public hospitals face this challenge. (Singh, HR)

Aware of its precarious position given staff shortages and its need for highly skilled nurses, CH has invested in sophisticated recruitment strategies.

Salaries

The salaries of public-sector hospital nurses are low compared with their counterparts in the private sector and internationally (see Table 2). Public-sector hospital nurses earn roughly two-thirds the pay of nurses in the private sector in South Africa (Thom, 2003). The same nurse working as a midwife in Saudi

Table 2. Nurses' Salaries in the Public Sector (per Month)

Nurse Level	Monthly wage (Rand)	Monthly wage (USD)[a,b]
Nurses on training (Std 8 level)	R2,641–R2,825	$283
Nurses on training (Std 10)	R3,033–R3,306	$331
Enrolled nursing assistants	R2,641–R3,306	$331
Senior nursing assistants	R3,560–R4,538	$454
Staff nurse	R3,560–R4,538	$454
Senior staff nurse	R5,214–R5,843	$585
Professional nurse	R5,214–R5,843	$585
Senior professional nurse	R6,494–R7,149	$715
Chief professional nurse	R8,066–R8,945	$895 ($10,740 yr)

[a]Rate of exchange 10:1, Rand to USD.
[b]Upper salary range

Arabia or medical ward nurse in the United Kingdom could earn more than four times what she would earn in a South African public hospital (Shevel, 2003). A public-sector staff nurse in South Africa earns the equivalent of around $7,000, compared with $40,000 for an equivalent job in the United States. An equivalent nurse (high-level professional) could earn $40,800 U.S. plus two plane tickets home per year in Saudi Arabia; $16,800 U.S. in the South African private sector; and $10,200 U.S. in the South African public sector. Salaries are bargained through a central labor council composed of representatives from all nursing unions at the national level.

Overseas Exodus

For managers at each hospital, nurses leaving for overseas jobs were the primary cause of the nursing shortage.[4] Managers at DH and RH reported that the current shortage and exodus of nurses overseas had begun in 1999–2000, and had worsened since. At all three hospitals nurses left for Saudi Arabia, primarily to be midwives, and for Great Britain, with lesser numbers going to the United States and Australia. Managers described that international recruitment was targeted at

[4]This was an unexpected finding. Although I was aware of shortages before visiting these hospitals and had read reports of international recruiting and brain drain, I did not expect to hear so much about these issues on the ground. Questions were designed to discuss the shortage; overseas emigration was an emerging topic.

professional skilled categories, though the nurse manager at DH indicated that nursing assistants and retired nurses were also actively recruited by the British firms.

> Saudi Arabia is taking our midwives. Of the five I mentioned (leaving), two are going to Saudi Arabia. (Ngubane, NM)

Managers were unanimous in the view that nurses left for financial reasons.

> It's a newer problem because people are going away. They are leaving for overseas, for Saudi Arabia, for better salaries. They lack green pastures. (Sizani, NM)

> Money is scarce in South Africa. There is no money. In the exit report, most list finances as the reason for leaving. The fact that nurses were offered an inadequate salary. . . . The problem with recruitment of nurses is at all levels. It's the salary, people don't want to work for this salary. (Mapley, HR)

> In 1999 nurses started to leave. It became worse in the year 2000. One of the biggest reasons is the debt, it affects them a lot. They are borrowing money from money lenders, then they face the pressure of trying to cope with their needs plus paying debts. (Sizani, NM)

> We have a problem with attrition. People are going overseas because of money. We don't have sufficient numbers of doctors, and we don't have sufficient numbers of nurses. (Ntsele, FM)

Recruiting

How to recruit and retain nurses in the context of the nursing shortage was an important topic for hospital managers. Given that they could not compete on salaries, they were limited by the advantages and disadvantages of their institutions. The competitive environment between public and private hospitals and among provincial hospitals, mattered, especially in attracting and keeping the most skilled nurses.

At DH, where the shortages were the most intense and prolonged, managers were not hopeful about their ability to attract new staff. Nurses at DH were compelled to live at the hospital due to lack of affordable accommodations nearby. Furthermore, there was little to entertain nurses; for a brief period the hospital had purchased DSTV (satellite television), but this had subsequently been forbidden by the DoH.

> In our business plan we identified the problem. People need entertainment, bureaucrats don't understand this. We had a DSTV, so people can watch TV, they have something to do. Now head office says we can't have it; but then they turn around and say, why are you not recruiting? (Ntsele, FM)

> It is not easy to recruit senior enrolled nurses, because most of them are interested in urban hospitals. Because here it is quiet, they don't have entertainment. So they always rush to go to the cities, where there are limelights and they can enjoy themselves. (Sizani, NM)

DH and the surrounding area lacked housing options:

> They don't want to share a room, but we cannot afford not to share. Everyone is here. The nearest town is Stanger, but there is absolutely no accommodation except for houses that go for half-a-million rand, but no rentals. Then many don't own a car. (Ndebele, HM)

The nurse manager described efforts to coordinate with nurse training programs to accept local applicants who could live at home and work at the hospital. Though hopeful that this might ease the shortage, she admitted that this was still 2 to 4 years off and that no local applicants had yet been contacted.

> A man from head office came, and we discussed the matter, and he advised me that I must write and ask for the creation of posts so that nurses could be promoted. So nothing happened. We opened entry-grade posts; so nothing happened. We advertised posts, nothing happened. We negotiated with training colleges to recruit some young ladies. We met with the superintendent general, and tried to increase intake. . . . We tried, they tried, nothing happened. So, with the help of the retired nurses, that is the only thing that has helped us to survive. They are very happy to come back, and it is nice to work with them. (Sizani, NM)

At RH, the nurse manager described what the hospital could offer:

> This is a very pleasant area to live, the climate is lovely, and we have excellent schools. These issues do tend to attract, but there isn't more I can offer. (West, HM)

In addition, she noted that the research possibilities presented by the poor population with high HIV prevalence might be attractive to young researchers. At the same time, the hospital manager lamented that there was nothing special she could offer in terms of salary, except to make sure that existing vacant posts were at the highest pay level for their classification.

> We have a really serious problem with recruitment of professional nurses. Recruitment and staffing issues have intensified. To recruit doctors and nurses to areas outside of Durban and Petermaritzburg is extremely difficult. . . . There is nothing special that I can offer in terms of salary, but we are trying to make sure that posts are senior enough to attract somebody; we make sure the salary is as high as we can get it. I would be very happy to support research that might attract a younger professional. There are thousands of research possibilities. We serve a very poor population, and we

have a high volume of HIV positive patients, and this would be of interest
to researchers with so much centering on HIV. (West, NM)

According to DoH rules, posts revert back to the entry level for that particular
classification. However, ranks could be upgraded if the hospital could successfully argue their need for an experienced staff under the "scarce skills" clause.[5]
Thus, RH sought to offer higher-ranked posts in hopes of attracting experienced
nurses from nearby hospitals whose experience qualified them. Everyone knew
this strategy simply "robbing Peter to pay Paul."

At CH, the nurse manager described how their recruitment strategy had been
carefully planned. She described commissioning a new hospital in the context
of the nursing shortage as the greatest challenge, but noted her hospital's comparative advantages in recruiting staff regionally.

> The biggest challenge has been commissioning a new hospital in the
> context of a shortage of nurses. The fact that it was a new hospital was
> an attraction. Its beautiful, you have accommodations in the form of the
> village, the residences are an attraction, especially for those coming from as
> far up as Johannesburg, coming from Eastern Cape, Northern Province.
> People could come knowing that there was accommodation. It has assisted
> us. (Mazibuko, NM)

Beyond its beautiful, new facility, subsidized accommodation, and proximity to
the "limelights" of Durban, CH benefited from additional recruiting resources. In
preparation for opening, the hospital held a widely publicized open house for
nurses. Staff collected names and phone numbers of nurses, who were later
contacted to discuss employment opportunities (Mazibuko, NM). No doubt this
well-organized strategy described by the nurse manager as "sensitizing people
toward this hospital," reached nurses in private and public sector employment.
Mazibuko concluded that these efforts helped to "front load" hiring, ensuring that
"by the time a new service is transferred, the nurses are there." At the same time,
hospital managers at CH admitted that as a tertiary/quaternary-care hospital,
they remained particularly vulnerable to shortages of nurses trained for theater
and ICU. Also, despite all of their advantages, CH failed to attract staff from the
decommissioned departments of other area hospitals, indicating that frequently
people want to remain in their jobs for a complex variety of reasons.

> We have two sources of staff. One source is from decommissioned hospitals.
> But staff have been reluctant to move for a variety of reasons. We have had to
> rely on recruiting. As we commission, we recruit. (Singh, HR)

---

[5]The "scarce skills" clause allows hospital-level human resources some leeway in, for
example, upgrading posts to attract staff with needed skills.

Rehiring Retirees

A key element of CH's recruitment strategy was rehiring retired nurses, some of whom were contacted through the open-house process. When CH prepared to open in 1999, management needed to secure a large complement of highly skilled nurses, especially highly skilled nurses for specialized medical and surgical services, in the context of a provincewide nursing shortage and low salaries. They projected that a good portion of their needs would be met through the movement of nurses from hospitals where services were decommissioned to the new hospital. However, as just stated, staff have been "reluctant to move for a variety of reasons" (Singh, HR). Hospital management then negotiated with the DoH to alter policy and allow retired nurses to be brought back on a contract basis.

At the time of this study, a full 12.5% of the nursing staff, 110 nurses, were rehired retirees. As the Occupational Health Nurse observed,

> Here they looked at the number of beds and nurses, and they resorted to employing retired nurses. If the retired nurses were not there, the shortage here would be more obvious. (Zuma, OHS)

Once this policy was altered to cope with the opening of the central hospital, other hospitals sought permission to rehire retirees. Each hospital offers different versions of the contract work based their situation. At CH, retired nurses are offered a yearly contract. At DH, nurses are also hired back on a yearly basis. The nurse manager described initiating the process to renew contracts 4 months in advance to allow ample time for the frequently slow DoH process. Presumably, this was to ensure that there would be no employment lapse. The nurse manager underscored the value of returned nurses many times during our interview:

> So, with the help of the retired nurses, that is the only thing that has helped us to survive. They are very happy to come back, and it is nice to work with them. They aren't getting much on their pension, that is another factor. (Sizani, NM)

At RH, retired nurses are hired for part-time schedules on monthly contracts so that they can easily be replaced if permanent staff is found.

> We are using retired nurses. We have changed posts around to attract them for 20 hours per week. Some work 8 to12, some 1 to 4. Five posts were converted, and we have 10 retired nurses at the moment. (Ngubane, NM)

Hospital managers expressed great satisfaction with the retired nurse's skill levels and dedication. At CH, managers noted that the computer courses and subsequent use of technology was especially challenging for older nurses. But no particular problems had emerged distinct from the general problems associated with the goal of going paperless. Hospital managers also noted that many who came back to work did so for financial reasons; nurses were not surviving well on a pension.

> They say there isn't much they get on retirement. Especially those that live in urban areas, they basically were really struggling. So they get some relief (by returning to work). (Sizani, HM)

> When we advertise, they come. Maybe we aren't preparing them for retirement, they don't have the resources. Maybe we need retirement preparation early enough to help people put more into retirement. (Ngubane, NM)

One financial factor that may be influencing older nurses work decisions is the fact that, similar to the crack epidemic in the United States, the HIV/AIDS epidemic is leaving older women as the caregivers for orphaned grandchildren, as well as potential breadwinners for a larger number of family members.

Work Organization Changes to Cope with Shortages

In at least one department at RH, altering work organization was explored as a means of coping with shortages. There, lower-ranked maternity department staff was trained to do tasks previously done by nurse midwives, so that the nurse midwife would be free to attend to births and focus on the things that she alone could do. The nurse manager, Mrs. Ngubane, admitted that this change required a "mind shift."

> Its going to be a mind shift. We must first get nurses together, firstly the maternity staff. Talk them over to this, show them what is happening. We need to talk to them, motivate them, get their minds to shift. I think if we start preparing them, let them buy in, it will work. (Ngubane, NM)

Experience of the "de-skilling" of select nursing tasks has been part of reducing labor costs in hospital reengineering efforts in developed countries.[6] While shifting tasks from a trained experience midwife to another nurse who might not have this preparation might be workable or desirable, there are probably ramifications (an experienced nurse might notice signs of complications, for example) for the loss of patient contact with the experienced nurse-midwife, even if the tasks that are part of that contact are rudimentary. Despite these international experiences, it is possible to see how task-shifting is practical, but how it could set dangerous precedents for staffing, care, and top-down decision making that could alienate nurses.

---

[6]Arguments against the fragmentation of nurses work into discrete tasks have included examples of how seemingly mundane aspects of care are opportunities for nurses to observe and evaluate patients during the hospital stay, and how lower-ranked nurses have been coerced into performing duties that they are not entirely trained for.

Absences

Another recent study of a district hospital in KZN found a high number of nurse absences and correlated this with the context of HIV/AIDS (showing an increase during the explosion of the epidemic) as a way to consider the impact of HIV/AIDS on nurses and the intensified workload of hospital nurses (Unger & Wells, 2002). I was not able to gather meaningful data from the hospitals on absences because of the way that records were kept. At DH, the nurse manager reported that absence was not a problem.

> Absenteeism isn't really a problem. We don't have much problem with alcohol or drugs, because nurses are too tired, they are overworked. They can't give their services to another institution. (Sizani, NM)

RH and CH related absenteeism to moonlighting and to the increased effects of HIV on nurses.

> We seem to have high levels of absenteeism on weekends and the night shift. On the other hand, it is impossible for us to keep track. We have a swiping system, but people refuse to swipe. So, ward managers record absences. My own thinking is that we must take into account that there is a shortage of nurses. But I don't know why there are absences. (Singh, HR)

Informally on tour, nurses and hospital personnel at CH and RH told me that nurses were frequently absent for 1 day in order to moonlight or because they had moonlighted and were resting. These short absences do not require a doctor's note and are not kept track of in a comprehensive way. They resulted in other nurses "picking up the slack."

The nurse manager at RH did an informal poll of the previous months' excused absences and suspected that many were related to HIV infection, judging by the ailments noted, especially increased TB among staff.

> Nurses themselves are sick or becoming sick. So there is more absenteeism, and that places more stress on the few others that are left. (West, NM)

> The HIV epidemic is taking a toll on our staff. Last month, I looked at how many were off sick, and I looked at the trends of who was off sick, and the ailments. Many had symptoms pointing to HIV. Two to three staff a month have gotten TB, young ones. This is also an indication of HIV infection. And a few have died, where the symptoms point in that direction. Last month, 46 nurses were off sick. These are documented illnesses lasting 3 days or more. (Ngubane, NM)

Moonlighting

In addition to seeking work overseas, managers at RH and CH indicated that moonlighting, though expressly forbidden by DoH policy, was a common practice.

> Most people are moonlighting to supplement. They want to get more money. (Zuma, OHS)

> There are shortages in the whole public service, but nurses work harder than other employees. People are forced to work overtime because of the shortage. We pay out a lot of overtime. This impacts people's health because they are working harder. (Singh, HR)

Nurse Staffing and Shortages: They "Lack Green Pastures" and Money

Shortages characterized the nursing labor market in KZN, but were experienced somewhat differently in each setting, depending on the facility's competitive advantage in recruiting staff. This fact links the settings of these three hospitals to the effects of nursing shortages on staffing. Hospitals that could offer better working conditions, even apart from salaries, held regional advantages in the competition for scarce staff.

Low salaries were identified as the cause of the nursing shortage. Overseas migration was a primary contributor to shortages, and nurses migrate for financial reasons. Financial problems also pushed retired nurses back into hospital work, and made moonlighting a common practice. The financial squeeze, exacerbated by neoliberal policies that increased unemployment and constrained health spending and the concurrent rise in prices for housing and food[7] pushed labor shortage dynamics.

Occupational Health Services

South Africa has a sophisticated occupational health policy that has been updated to reflect the occupational risks associated with HIV/AIDS.

As foundation for understanding, I summarize workplace policies and practices on which nurses and managers commented most extensively.

---

[7] In 2002 the food price index rose 17%, while nonfood inflation rose 7%. The price of maize meal, the staple of the diet of the poor and working class in South Africa, doubled in 2002. The working class spends one-third of its income on food, the poor spend one-half of their income on food (Watkinson & Makgetla, 2002). Trends in housing costs and values are also on the rise, except for the houses of the poor and working class, which lag behind in value.

South Africa's National Occupational Health Policy

South Africa's national occupational health policy includes safe needle disposal and reporting of bloodborne pathogen exposure (Republic of South Africa, 1993); antiretroviral post-exposure prophylaxis (PEP) (Republic of South Africa, 2000), and compensation for workers who contract HIV and other bloodborne diseases at work (RSA, 1993) (see Box 1). Occupational health policy is made at the national level, dictated through the provincial Department of Health (DoH) and implemented within hospitals. The provincial DoH is also the employer for the provincial public health system.

Post-Exposure Prophylaxis Protocol (RSA, 1999)

Following an accidental exposure to blood, the established protocol instructs health workers to clean the wound properly and take a "stat dose" of zidovudine

---

Box 1: South African Occupational Health Policy on Workplace Exposure to HIV/AIDS

General Occupational Health and Safety Protection and Compensation
- Occupational Health and Safety Act (OHSA), 1993
- Compensation for Occupational Injuries and Diseases Act (COIDA), 1993

Safe Sharps Disposal and Personal Protective Equipment
- Hazardous Biological Agents Regulations, Occupational Health and Safety Act (OSHA), 1993

Post-Exposure Prophylaxis (PEP) and Workers' Compensation for HIV/AIDS[†]
- Code of Good Practice: Key Aspects of HIV/AIDS and Employment (2000)
  Labor Relations Act, 1995; Employment Equity Act, 1998
- Management of Occupational Exposure to the Human Immunodeficiency Virus (HIV), (1999)

[†]Antiretroviral PEP is available in provincial hospitals. To obtain PEP employee is required to have an HIV test in order to determine whether HIV infection predates workplace exposure. If employee is found to already be HIV+, PEP is ceased. This procedure is intended to prevent unnecessary ARV/PEP treatment and to establish culpability of workplace exposure in HIV infection.

Reprinted by permission from Macmillan Publishers Ltd: Jennifer Zelnick and Max O'Donnell, The Impact of the HIV/AIDS Epidemic on Hospital Nurses in KwaZulu Natal, South Africa: Nurses' Perspectives and Implications for Health Policy, *Journal of Public Health Policy, 26,* 163-185, copyright 2005. Published by Palgrave Macmillan.

(AZT) and lamivudine (3TC) for post-exposure prophylaxis. If the patient whose blood was the source of the exposure agrees to be tested, the hospital or clinic administers a "rapid test" for HIV. If the source patient does not consent to be tested, he or she is treated as HIV positive. If confirmed negative by test, PEP for the exposed worker is ceased; If confirmed positive by test, the hospital issues the health worker a 1-month supply of PEP. According to the protocol, the health worker must be tested following an injury; those who refuse testing do not qualify for PEP. Refusal also "negates any future claim with respect to the injury." If the health worker tests positive, the protocol calls for the worker to "stop the drugs, counsel, and plan for future management." Only health workers who consent to a test, and test negative on a rapid test and lab test, receive full PEP treatment.

Workers are required to report injuries to a supervisor within an hour and to complete an "injury on duty" form for transmission to the compensation commissioner. Workers who are able to establish that their HIV infection is due to an incident at work are entitled to compensation as outlined in the 1993 Compensation for Occupational Injuries and Diseases Act (COIDA). A November 19, 2004, draft amendment to COIDA specifies compensation for occupationally acquired HIV/AIDS, and access to antiretroviral treatment is explicitly guaranteed as a compensated Medical-Aide benefit (RSA, 2004). Up to this date, medical treatment was generally guaranteed, though ARV treatment was not specified.

South Africa's National Department of Health adopted one of three PEP courses recommended by the U.S. Public Health Service (PHS) in 2001 (Centers for Disease Control, 2001; RSA, 1999). This regime includes two reverse transcriptase inhibitors, zidovudine (AZT) and lamivudine (3TC). The 2001 South African guidelines also recommend that the protease inhibitor indinivir be added to AZT/3TC in the event of very high risk exposures (as determined by the nature of the exposure and the viral load of the source patient). In 1998 the AZT/3TC combination was the recommended course under PHS guidelines. The PHS subsequently updated these guidelines in 2001 because new data suggested mutations associated with ZDV and 3TC resistance might be common in some areas; new drugs from the same family as indinivir were also recommended for three-drug combinations in the updated guidelines because of possible resistance. South African national guidelines have not been revised to reflect 2001 PHS updates.

Antiretroviral agents are associated with adverse side effects, including nausea, diarrhea, and headaches (CDC, 2001). Data from the U.S. National Surveillance System for Health Care Workers and the HIV Post-exposure Prophylaxis Registry indicate that nearly 50% of U.S. health care personnel report adverse events while taking PEP, and about one third stop taking the drugs as a result (Gerberding, 2003). Serious adverse events are rare in a 4-week course of PEP, but they do occur and can be life threatening.

Precautions

South Africa's DoH requires hospital nurses to follow universal precautions: wear gloves for all contacts with body fluid (CDC, 1987); treat each patient as if HIV positive; properly dispose of needles in secure disposal boxes; and never recap or dislodge used needles from the syringe, previously a routine practice. (In KZN a company specializing in medical waste properly disposes of needles.)

HIV Status: Confidentiality

Confidentiality of patient HIV status is a common practice that is enshrined in multiple policies. The HIV/AIDS policy of the South African Nursing Council, the body that oversees licensing of all nurses, states that patients have "a right to confidentiality" (SANC, 1999). The 1990 Department of Health National Policy on Testing for HIV (RSA, 1990), now incorporated into the 2000 Department of Health's National Policy on Testing for HIV (RSA, 2000), states that "the information regarding the result of the test must remain fully confidential, and may only be disclosed in the absence of an overriding legal or ethical duty with the individual's fully informed consent." Health worker confidentiality is also specifically referred to in the PEP policy requiring hospitals to assign health workers a number and keep test results confidential (KZN, 2001).

KZN Protocol Following Workplace Blood Exposure (KZN, 2001)

1. *Immediate attention to the wound*
   This includes squeezing out blood and cleaning with soap and water.
2. *Reporting the injury*
   This includes reporting the injury to the appropriate manager for the purpose of initiating both the PEP process and the paperwork that is required for each injury. Reporting allows the nurse to access PEP, and the hospital to keep track of the occurrence of needlesticks and use this information for education and prevention. Paperwork for hospital records is typically filled out with the manager who handles the occupational health program; workers compensation paperwork is typically filled out with the human resources manager and forwarded to the DoH. Unreported injuries are not eligible for compensation from the government.
3. *Voluntary Counseling and Testing (VCT)*
   VCT refers to the way that testing is delivered; nurses' are supposed to be counseled pre- and post-test by a trained HIV counselor. Nurses must consent to testing in order to be eligible for PEP and workers compensation. Patients are also offered VCT if their HIV status is unknown in order to determine the risk level of the injury and to decide whether or not PEP is indicated. If the source patient refuses to be tested, the highest level of risk is assumed. The nurses' refusal to be tested ends the process of PEP and WC.

4. *PEP treatment with a ARV drugs*

At the time of reporting, after consenting to VCT, the nurse is given a stat dose of AZT and 3TC. In the event of a very high risk exposure, a third drug (indinavir) is added to the regimen. If the rapid test comes back positive, no further PEP is given. If the rapid test is negative, blood is drawn for the Eliza test, which is sent to the lab, and the nurse is given a prescription for 2 weeks of PEP drugs. If the second test comes back positive, PEP is ceased. A positive result at either point indicates that the nurse was already infected with HIV at the time of the injury. A negative result indicates that the nurse should continue PEP, and a second prescription is given for the final 2 weeks of the short-course treatment. Monitoring is expected to be done when the second prescription is obtained.

5. *Follow up testing and counseling*

Follow-up tests are done at 3, 6, and 12 months. If the nurse is found positive at a later point, and PEP protocol was followed, it is assumed that the workplace exposure led to infection and the process for workers compensation continues.

OHS in the Three Hospitals

Although the topic of occupational health and occupational health services was introduced broadly, the managers interviewed focused on needlesticks and workplace transmission of HIV as their chief concern. This indicated that HIV infection was seen as the primary occupational health risk. The second-most-frequently discussed health issue, typically related to comments about HIV/AIDS and staff shortages, was stress.

The most striking thing about the OHS services at these three hospitals is the difference in the level of services offered, especially in the numbers and skills of dedicated personnel. This undoubtedly has repercussions for how the services are utilized by nurses, and ultimately for the occupational health of staff. However, despite the significant differences described in this section, comments by hospital managers about reporting, accidental injuries, and nurse utilization of OHS services are strikingly similar. They describe an attitude toward HIV/AIDS— whether in patients or staff—that is characterized by stigma and denial that had huge impacts on the programs in place to protect nurses. A preliminary conclusion supported by these findings is that, while better OHS services could improve staff occupational health, stigma and denial of HIV/AIDS were more important in determining critical program elements such as reporting, VCT, and PEP.

Comparison between OHS at the Three Hospitals

Occupational health and safety for provincial hospitals is overseen at the provincial level by the deputy director of occupational health. Since the formation of KZN in 1994, the post of deputy director for OH was filled for 1 year, and then vacant for 8 years. In May 2003 a new director of occupational health was hired. While not too much was made of this gap in management of occupational health, the hospital manager at DH described occupational health at the provincial level as in a "formative stage" (Ndebele, HM). The occupational health nurse at CH noted that, while the lack of authority gave her more room to follow her own initiative, it robbed her of authority in the bureaucratic environment.

> It would help if we had policies and procedures from the DoH. This hasn't been given, such as, you need to base your program on this. I have given my program to King Edward and Addington. This is all supposed to be under the deputy director for occupational health, he just started. You need to know the department's goals to function. You rely on previous experience to apply here, but you cannot get cooperation if the dictate is not from management. You always get the question, "Does department know about this?" (Zuma, OHS)

At DH, there is no occupational health clinic and no trained occupational health nurse. Mrs. Megeba, a ward nurse, heads the occupational health and safety committee, which is charged with dealing with all OHS issues. Mrs. Megeba felt inadequate in her position due to the demands of her work on the wards in the short-staffed hospital:

> There is no support from outside. It is very difficult for me, dealing with health and safety, because I am full-time on the wards. I am not managing well. I am the chairperson for health and safety, but much of the time I spend on the wards, and this side is neglected. (Megeba, OHS)

Additionally, an infection-control nurse handles education and issues related to infections in the hospital, including worker exposures. Recently the province initiated training to promote the formation of EAP programs at provincial hospitals. There is an employee assistance program at DH that has resources for staff health, and there are trained HIV counselors that are available for staff as well as patients.

Mrs. Megeba described health education as "what the hospital has in place to protect nurses from needlesticks."

> Nurses learn about the safe disposal of the needles and the proper disposal of the buckets and the way we handle the needles. Education is going on now and then. If any nurse is involved in a needlestick, there is a protocol for how to protect the person from being infected with HIV. (Megeba, OHS)

Health education at DH consists of twice-a-month sessions given on the wards by the infection-control nurse (Megeba, OHS). The system for disposal of used needles and protocol following needlestick incidents were described as key components of health education.

The protocol following a needlestick is the same in all provincial hospitals to the extent that it is dictated by the requirements of workers compensation policy and post-exposure prophylaxis policy. However, the details of how this policy is implemented vary by hospital based on the facilities and personnel available. Problems of confidentiality were noted as key criticisms of the program.

> This is the only place in the area where a person can get tested. Except for private, but not near here. (Dlamini, SW)

Another issue is needle disposal. DH, like RH, used plastic disposal buckets for used needles. Disposal buckets are kept on an injection cart along with all supplies. Buckets are picked up weekly by Compass Waste, a medical waste disposal company based in KZN. Problems related to needle disposal are discussed further in the sections below; the hospital manager characterizes the problem in general as the lack of "importance" assigned to the disposal bins.

> One thing that has actually happened is that people do not assign importance to the disposal containers, and there was a time when they were emptied into open areas. Now they are kept in the wards and picked up by this company, Compass. But the infection-control nurse will tell you that this is not ideal, she needs a locked space, which takes us bask to our issue of space shortage. (Ndebele, NM)

One aspect of the occupational health program that seemed functional at DH was the EAP. The committee, composed of a union and an HR representative, two nurses and a social worker, reported dealing with numerous staff concerns. Ms. Dlamini, the social worker, an engaging young, energetic woman, reported that nurses were "comfortable coming to me because they know I am a social worker." Also trained as an HIV/AIDS counselor, the presence of this social worker could be an asset for nurses seeking HIV/AIDS advice. Some studies have found that nurses prefer to be counseled by people they perceive to be of equal ranks to themselves (Holt, MD). The social worker demonstrated good knowledge of AIDS treatment issues, and described her intention of focusing on treatment literacy with nursing staff.

At RH, like DH, occupational health services were run by a nurse with no formal OH background. However, unlike services at DH, there was an office for occupational health and safety, and the sister in charge did not have ward duties (though she did manage decontamination, which was her area of expertise). She had held the post for less than a year, and she replaced a Sister Richards, who had built up the health and safety program with education and very good record-keeping methods. Sister Richards' work provided the basic infrastructure for health and safety services. Despite the accolades for Sister Richards' work, the nurse manager with less than a year seniority had this perception of the program at RH:

> Health and safety hasn't been a priority. We don't really have the structure. We don't have a qualified occupational nurse. The one doing health and safety is just one of the nurses. (Ngubane, NM)

Another new staff member, the infection-control nurse, had these recommendations:

> They need a staff clinic and an occupational sister. Striker is doing health and safety, but she isn't an occupational nurse. They need someone who is dedicated to staff health. (White, ICN)

One specific problem with the implementation of needlestick protocol at RH concerned confidentiality. Like DH, hospital managers referred to the size of the hospital and nurses appearance at the casualty department after a needlestick. The limited hours of the infection-control nurse seemed to add confusion and hassle to the process. As she explained,

> I don't think that everybody is happy about the confidentiality. I am only here 8 to12. If I am not here, they have to wait. And when I am here, I am often out in the hospital. (White, ICN)

Asked to explain what the hospital had in place to protect nurses from accidental exposures to potentially HIV infected blood, the RH hospital manager explained,

> We have everything in place to prevent needlestick injuries. They have the possibility of safe disposal, we have strict control over the disposing of medical waste, they are given gloves to protect themselves, midwives and nurses in theater are provided with goggles and clothing, but there is a huge reluctance from the providers themselves to make use. To get compliance with policies, to get people to comply is a major, major area. (West, HM)

The issue of nurse compliance with OHS policy presents a dynamic in which OHS policies are rules to be followed, not programs in which nurses are active, empowered participants.[8]

Hospital managers described in-service training and the orientation for new staff as the key components of occupational health education for nurses. The infection-control nurse described an upcoming in-service training in English and Zulu, and said that in her opinion these trainings should occur four times per year. At the same time, she was critical of the effectiveness of these training courses:

---

[8] For example, the RH has a five-part procedure for reporting employee failure to use personal protective equipment, which can lead to disciplinary action, and enlists the health and safety representative as an "enforcer."

> They have had training with Sister Richards last year. But I don't know how many it gets across to. I haven't had any nurse incidents, not many anyway. Three of the 33 or 34 were nurses. Nursing sisters are well-informed, but a staff nurse who was injured was ignorant (she didn't know the risk. Though she knew the transmission routes, she didn't know the treatment side effects). (White, ICN)

> Training on occupational health, HIV, and disposal is covered in the orientation for new staff, including doctors. But people tend to listen, not ask questions during training. They are not tested and evaluated on their knowledge. I attended a week-long orientation myself when I first came. People just sit there, they don't ask questions. I don't know if this is a problem with culture, where people tend not to argue, talk back, or ask. I was asking questions all the time, but I've been brought up to argue, and I think a lot of the black staff haven't. (White, ICN)

Again, as at DH, proper disposal of used needles and waste disposal were noted as problem areas. The buckets were identified as "not solid enough," and the occupational health sister demonstrated how easy it was to pop open a sealed bucket. Both the infection-control and occupational health sisters indicated that they were aware that a better bucket was available, but it was unclear what steps if any had been taken to obtain better equipment. At the same time, hospital managers only indicated problems with improper disposal, not equipment failure of the buckets. The hospital manager indicated that measures had been taken to address disposal problems, including posters in the wards, checking trash bags, and even threatening nurses that they are breaking the law when they improperly dispose of needles.

> We have sensitized two health and safety representatives from each area. There has been in-service training, lots and lots. At every departmental heads meeting, we've encouraged them to check bags before they leave the wards, trying to sensitize people to the presence of a needle in the bag. There are policies on disposal of sharps, and we have distributed a poster to put up in the areas where the sharps are disposed of that shows correct procedure. (West, HM)

> We have very advanced health and safety legislation. According to this legislation, it's unlawful to put yourself or anybody else in danger. Even that hasn't made a difference, but it might be part of our orientation in the coming year. (West, HM)

The hospital manager explained that the new deputy director of occupational health from provincial DoH had advanced the position that it is actually unlawful according to occupational health legislation to "put yourself or anybody else in danger." This interpretation of national policy from management's perspective portrays the policy as punitive—negatively focused on nurses' behavior.

Unlike DH, the EAP program at RH seemed not to function particularly effectively. The reason given by management was that EAP officers were white, and black staff did not trust them to advance their interests. An interview with one of the EAP representatives, a white male, showed him to be entirely insensitive to this issue.[9] At the same time, the health and safety committee was functioning, with two representatives appointed from each area.

The infection-control nurse, who had worked for Anglo American[10] in their staff clinic, believed that a staff clinic at the hospital would be of huge benefit for the occupational health program in general, and needlestick-related programs in particular. She noted that staff clinics were absent in health care, and that the public sector could use industry as a model for these services.

At CH, the occupational health clinic is staffed and run by a trained occupational health nurse with extensive experience in private-sector industry. The OHS services at CH are highly organized and include the clinic, a large representative health and safety committee, and a separate safety department. Infection control is less involved in occupational issues than at other hospitals in this study. Since the central labs for the province are located at CH, access to blood tests and results is swifter than at other hospitals. With the entire hospital computerized, there is a good system for confidentiality of test results. Finally, the size of the hospital also aids confidentiality since people's comings and goings are not so easily observed.

There is an open management position to supervise the clinic, and there is a staff assistant present. The clinic handles screening for the large complement of staff, as well as coordinating education and handling all aspects of occupational health and safety. At the time of this study, the large health and safety committee was preparing for its second meeting.

The occupational health nurse described how needlestick protocol is implemented at CH:

> We've got policies, it's in the system, and everyone knows about it. If you are injured, you must report immediately to your supervisor. Do first-aid, squeeze under water and clean. The supervisor must sit with the person, and if here is a doctor in the ward, they sit together and explain— we must take your blood, blood of the source patient, and so on. It's up to you, there is an indemnity that you sign, that you agree or don't agree. (Zuma, OHS)

> If it is 7 to 4 they come here to the clinic, if 4 to 6, they go to the domain manager. If it is night, they go to the night domain. (Zuma, OHS)

[9] Interview not included in this analysis.

[10] Anglo American is a multinational corporation that began in South Africa gold mining. Gold mines are still its primary presence in SA.

> You must do the testing here. There is a lot of confidentiality. The system saves us. You use the KZN admit number, and no one can get the results but me. The system is very secure and anonymous. (Zuma, OHS)

> When you come here to the clinic, everyone knows that if you have a stick you must have a test, but no one knows if you agree to the test or not. (Zuma, OHS)

> Initially we try to introduce social worker/psychologist, to prepare for a later stage. So they know it doesn't end with the occupational health nurse, it will go further. You still emphasize that even if it goes to that person, confidentiality will be maintained. (Zuma, OHS)

> People come in with an upset stomach on the PEP drugs, and I tell them, don't take the drugs in the day, eat something and take them at night. Many finish with no problem. (Zuma, OHS)

Discussing the program at CH, comfortably seated in one of the rooms in the staff clinic, Zuma's level of knowledge on all aspects of OHS services was apparent. Furthermore, her explanations of handling nurses' anxieties and the practicalities following a needlestick revealed a deep comfort level with discussing the issues and taking appropriate actions. Zuma was a skilled professional with a developed interest in preventing and managing occupational illness and injury. This was a marked contrast to the other hospitals piecemeal programs.

In addition, equipment was different at CH than at the other sites. CH had disposal bins made of hard plastic (see Figure 1). Rather than a bucket design (see Figure 2), disposal bins of hard plastic where the nurse or doctor laid the needle horizontally into a slot, and then shut the cover causing the needle to roll into the bin, were in use. While the bins were still kept on injection carts, the hospital was looking into mounting these onto the wall as is the practice in U.S. facilities. These containers were chosen after a comparison of available options. At CH, a "needleless" catheter system for the ICU was also in the process of adoption. The domain system, in which departments have budgetary discretion, facilitated the procurement of the superior equipment. It is likely that the fact of setting up a new facility also allowed for innovations in ordering. Still, the contrast between CH and the other hospitals is clear.

It is worth pointing out that, despite the superior program infrastructure and equipment, the OHS staff at CH made the following observation:

> My assessment is that nurses have got all the knowledge as far as the virus, transmission, and management. But when it comes to the workplace, I don't know whether it is pressure of work or whatever. But on the needlestick injury, when you look at them, there is no injury that you can justify that she "couldn't do anything," that it had to happen. Our assumption is negligence in most cases. KZN is the province in SA with the highest rate of HIV, so you would think everyone is more conscious about the needlestick and blood.

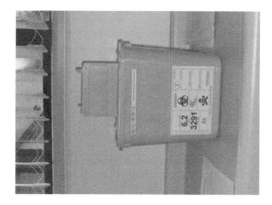

Disposal buckets RH.

Disposal bin CH.

Figure 1. Disposal bins for used needles from RH and CH. Photographs by author.

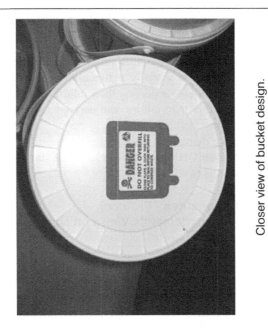

Closer view of bucket design.

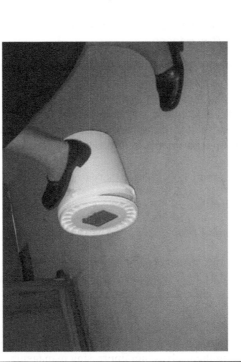

Nurse demonstrates flimsy bucket.

Figure 2. Closer view of RH disposal buckets.
Photographs by author.

> We are disappointed that from July 2002 until now, we have had 3 or 4
> reported each month. (Zuma, OHS)

One thing that is supported by other situations is the fact that the higher level
of reported needlesticks is actually a function of the better program, where
more people are comfortable reporting their injuries. This higher rate should be
taken as a success rather than failure, and perhaps an indication of the level of
underreporting in other facilities.

To summarize, the disparities between hospital settings described in part one
had a lot of bearing on OHS programs in terms of staff, space, equipment, and
confidentiality systems (see Table 3).

Workplace HIV Exposures: Protocol, Prevention, and Management's Views on Nurses

Reported Needlestick Injuries

Needlestick injuries were described as underreported by both managers and
nurses. Further, the official data provided by infection control was frequently
contradicted by statements from management. However, Table 4 shows that the
extremely underdeveloped system at DH resulted in far fewer reported injuries.

Needlestick Injuries: Management's Perspective on How and Why They Happen

Hospital managers reported that giving injections, suturing, and improper
disposal (including leaving the needle lying on the bed or putting it in the
waste bin), and the practice of recapping were the most common reasons for
needlestick injury. Negligence, carelessness, and noncompliance were terms that
hospital managers used to describe the cause of needlestick injuries. This is a
common perspective on the cause of needlestick injuries, as well as most other
occupational injury.

At RH, the nurse manager reported that casualty nurses were the most exposed.

> Casualty nurses are mostly exposed. We see a lot of trauma, people come
> in bleeding from domestic violence, gunshots. They are handling a lot of
> blood. (Ngubane, NM)

At the same time, managers' assessments of carelessness were sympathetic.
For example, at DH, the hospital manager noted that if needlesticks were the
result of "nurse's carelessness, then management needs to put something in
place." At RH, the hospital manager cited "denial" and the fact that "we are so
close to the disease" as equally important in explaining nurse failure to follow
protocol, and the nurse manager focused on the need for nurses to understand that
they are protecting themselves, not impressing management for following rules.

Table 3. Comparison of OHS at Three Hospitals

Hospitals	Staff	Space		OHS programs				
			Education	Equipment	EAP	OHS committee	Confidentiality
DH	None dedicated or trained (plus IC, not present for interview)	None	Twice per month by ICN	Thin disposal buckets, lack of storage	Good	Good, handles all OHS issues	Systems for privacy, problems in practice
RH	One dedicated, untrained (plus ICN)	Desk and files in decontamination room	Various formats, NM, and ICN	Thin disposal buckets	Poor	OK	Systems for privacy, problems in practice
CH	Two dedicated and trained (plus ICN)	Clinic with two private rooms	Sophisticated schedule for education plus on-line training	Quality disposal bins, some needleless systems	Not yet	Highly organized, in infancy	Highly private, computerized only OHS nurse can obtain results

Table 4. Reported Needlestick
Injuries for 2002-2003 at
Three Hospitals

Hospital	Number of reported needlestick injuries May 2002–May 2003
DH	2
RH	32
CH	34

You find that in the wards, universal precautions are everywhere. But you just find them recapping, they just recap needles, they reject precautions. Investigating a needlestick, when you follow through, and find them trying to recap a needle in this day and age! How can you do that? Only when you come for rounds, they will quickly put on gloves to impress you. And you say, no, don't impress us. It's your life. You've got to protect yourself and the patients. We've got to protect each other. (Ngubane, NM)

Still, management expressed frustration with negligence and noncompliance, and their words contradict other impulses to present policy as nonpunitive and supportive.

Six weeks ago I was attacked by a swarm of bees, and admitted here for my care. The nurse was putting up an IV therapy on me without gloves. I asked why was she not wearing gloves, and she said she couldn't put up the drip with gloves. I said, "But you don't know my HIV status." Even when I tried to motivate, "Please go put on gloves" she said, "Nei nei nei, I won't put on gloves, I can't do the IV with gloves on." So we've not succeeded in changing habits. When Mr. Mbaso came to our committee last week, we had him highlight that it is actually unlawful to dispose of sharps in the bin. (West, HM)

Last year there were 33 or 34 needlestick injuries, 3 or 4 a month. They occur because of negligence and inadequate disposal. (White, ICN)

On the needlestick injuries, when you look at them, there is no injury that you can justify that she "couldn't do anything," that it had to happen. Our assumption is negligence in most cases. KZN is the province in SA with the highest rate of HIV, so you would think everyone is more conscious about the needlestick and blood. We are disappointed that from July 2002 until now, we have had 3 or 4 reported each month. (Zuma, OHS)

Both DH and RH had had recent injuries involving needlesticks that were caused by improper disposal.

> We have stopped putting the container outside, people just empty the container in the plastic garbage. The man who comes to collect was pricked. This is such a problem because then there is nobody to test, just a used needle. (Sizani, NM)

There were contradictions between what hospital managers told me and their own views and actions, although capturing this was extremely limited due to single interviews and short visits. Still, this suggests some of the realities underneath policy implementation in the provincial hospital environment. At RH, in contrast to the nurse manager's frustration over the practice of recapping needles—a practice forbidden by universal precautions—a matron who had acted as nurse manager demonstrated how to use the top of the needle disposal bucket to dislodge the needle from the syringe prior to disposal. Presumably this was the former practice, but the fact that a figure of authority within the hospital was unaware of the change was disconcerting.

The nurse manager at DH described her own failure to report a needlestick, and her belief that nurses did not become HIV+ through patient contact.

> I don't think they get HIV through patient contact. Nobody has been positive after a needlestick. They get it the normal way that people get it. (Sizani, NM)

Though her view is borne out by known figures on the incidence of seroconversion after occupational injury, it could still undermine current protocols.

Reporting, Voluntary Counseling and Testing (VCT), and Post-Exposure Prophylaxis (PEP) and Workers Compensation (WC)

The protocol following a needlestick injury has several components. Among these are ones aimed at preventing an accidental exposure from becoming an HIV infection; those aimed at counseling the injured worker; and those that are part of establishing the workplace origin of infection.[11]

Hospital managers at all three hospitals described many problems with the components of this system. They agreed, for example, that nearly all those who reported needlestick injuries were HIV negative.

> I would imagine injuries are underreported. Most of the people who report are HIV negative. If someone knows their status, I don't think they will report whatsoever. Given infection rates, some staff must be infected. So the process isn't followed that well. (White, ICN)

---

[11] See pp. 105-106 of this section for protocol details.

> They know it is possible that they are HIV positive because they are having needlesticks, and they are having unprotected sex . . . it's possible they are HIV positive, they know it, that is why they are all so scared. It's only those who know there is this possibility who are scared to do the test, not those who know it's not possible. (Dlamini, DH)

> You will find that there is a person who has a needlestick who knows their status, that it is positive, so she doesn't want to subject herself to a test. (Zuma, OHS)

For managers, the negative HIV status of nurses who reported needlesticks was confirmation that those who knew—or suspected—that they were HIV+ did not report injuries. Among the reasons that hospital managers thought nurses did not report, especially those who suspected they could be HIV+, was denial (not wanting to have their status confirmed), fear of being talked about, and distrust of the system for confidentiality.

> At the same time that people have needlesticks, they don't want to report them. You can't trust people to report, but it would be nice if people took responsibility for their own health. Because it's not just about whether you are HIV negative or not, its also getting treatment and taking the necessary precautions. From the management side, that's the problem; but I don't know what the nurses would feel like. (Ndebele, HM)

> Sometimes they don't report. There are those who are afraid to take blood, to do the test, so they don't report. They are concerned about knowing there status, about everybody talking. They are not sure if it will be kept confidential. They don't come forward. (Megeba, OHS)

Hospital managers also indicated that not reporting injuries in the context where no treatment for the disease was offered was logical, especially with the stakes so high regarding stigmatization.

> They have good reasons not to report. If I know my status, why should I report? It won't change anything, I'll get a starter pack, the results will come back positive, and treatment will end. It's a stigma. If you have a needlestick injury, everyone will want to know, "Has Zuma had a test, what happened, how was your blood?" And if the patient's status is known, people will assume that the nurse is infected because the patient is full blown. (Zuma, OHS)

> They are very secretive, they don't come forward. Confidentiality is so much. Maybe we are not trustworthy. I do not know what the problem is, that they do not confide in management to say, I am HIV positive. Maybe because we cannot offer them anything, as far as ARV. (Ngubane, NM)

Hospital managers described a high level of denial about HIV/AIDS among nurses. They evidenced this denial by virtue of the fact that even those with Medical Aide that covered ARVs did not want to go on the drugs, and that even witnessing the death of patients, friends, and families did not motivate nurses to action.

> We still don't know how to penetrate this denial. We've been educating people, people are dying, each and everyone has someone close who is dead, but people still don't do anything about it. (Dlamini, SW)

The hospital manager at RH described how this denial spilled over into patient interactions, indicating that nurses possibly viewed such behavior as a practical part of coping.

> We've introduced questions and management related to HIV because of the huge problem of HIV in children. When you assess nurses that are using the approach, assessment after assessment, they avoid the HIV questions. And if you question it—a researcher at our poly-teknikon did research on why nurses avoided these questions—a common response was, "If I ask these questions a mother might think her child is HIV positive," and then if you ask if this is a bad thing they say yes, because if she thinks her child is HIV she will think that she is HIV positive, that will upset the mother, she will be depressed, and she won't be able to take care of herself and her baby. (West, HM)

The hospital manager described her view that health care providers often transferred their own fear of being positive onto patients.

> Health care providers are scared to discuss HIV/AIDS because they are scared that they cannot handle the emotions and all the complications. And then there is the fear of, perhaps I am HIV positive too. And how am I going to handle it? Because of the position of African women, they are not in a position to demand safe sex. She doesn't have the authority. And I don't know of any African woman that isn't living in fear of being infected. It's that same similar process of denial . . . yet they have free access to everything to prevent transmission on the job. (West, HM)

The social position of African women has been identified as a key contributor to an epidemic where numbers of women infected increasingly exceed that of men (UNAIDS, 2004). Long-time African public health practitioners have argued for putting resources into the development of protections for women such as the female condom and vaginal microbicide that did not rely on male consent (Susser, 2002). This is a direct acknowledgment of the intractable difficulties in changing sexual behavior and traditional relationships, at least quickly enough in the context of the rapid spread of HIV/AIDS. If true, the acknowledgement that all African women are living in fear of being infected, in the context of occupational exposure and reporting requirements, means that most nurses have a legitimate fear of reporting injuries and agreeing to VCT. West acknowledged denial as a mechanism for coping in this context, where nurses' knowledge of risk factors could not protect them from risk in their marriages/sexual partnerships. Hospital managers felt that nurses did not trust the confidentiality of test results, and that this presented another hindrance to VCT. Some managers indicated that this was more the result of the workplace "rumor mill" than actual lapses in the system.

> There is a system for confidentiality. But I don't know what goes wrong with the people who are handling it, because much of the time a person has done the test, then you hear rumors that so-and-so did it, and the results are this way. But because there are people who are actually doing the VCT and they are not involved. They are the only person who knows about the result and everything. (Megeba, OHS)

> Nurses don't respect confidentiality for HIV/AIDS. Stigma and gossip prevent people from getting support of their colleagues. (Zuma, OHS)

At the same time, specific problems were observed, associated with the size of the hospital, visibility of testing places, and close working relationships between injured workers and those doing the tests.

> It's possible to know everything in the hospital. So they think there will be no confidentiality, although there is. It is also stressing for the person who is doing the test, because he meets this person everyday. They told me they have stress—they would rather not test the staff, because he or she will say that I have been telling that he has been tested, or that he is positive. I think this is because it is a very small hospital. I think in a bigger hospital, where there are different departments, it's not so easy to meet everyone from every department. (Dlamini, SW)

> I think the process is not good. It's a small hospital. Even though everyone uses codes and it's supposed to be confidential, but it goes to casualty, they have to walk over there in plain view, though they are given a code and see the doctor, in a closed room. (White, ICN)

Each hospital had different systems for confidentiality. At DH, confidentiality was the responsibility of those involved with implementing protocol. At RH, confidentiality of test results was maintained through the practice of limiting access to lab results to the infection-control nurse, who also happened to be white and socially removed from the other nurses. This policy created a different set of problems, since this nurse worked only limited hours (days 8 to 12), and was often difficult to locate around the hospital when at work. At CH, the system was very sophisticated because of access to a computer network. Results were stored anonymously, and only the OHS nurse had access to the code into the system.

Furthermore, the size of the institution, and full-time dedicated OHS staff were also advantages for confidentiality.

Dr. Holt at RH saw the government's failure to provide a confidential testing site away from the hospital as a key failure in their support and protection of the workforce. Holt was involved with an NGO in the area that delivered hospice care that initiated an off-site test when they realized that nurses wouldn't be comfortable being tested at a small workplace.

> At hospice, we knew that everyone would know if anyone tested, would know their status. So we put the whole process away from hospice, and then hospice agreed to fund ARV. I now have 1 or 2 staff on ARV. If the state could be more like that, like "We don't really need to know who you are, but we will pay." I really think the state doesn't go out of their way to value doctors and nurses. Not even a little confidential testing site, they don't give anything. (Holt, MD)

Hospital managers indicated that many nurses quit PEP because of side effects, and that nurses were aware of and fearful of these effects.

> There is a lot of noncompliance with PEP among staff. Once people start feeling sick, they stop taking it. We start with a 2 week script, and as soon as we know the p24 result, we cancel or refill, but usually the staff doesn't refill after the first script. (White, ICN)

> Nurses do not have enough information. If someone hears that these drugs cause reactions, then the other is also afraid of the reactions. They don't like this treatment. (Megeba, OHS)

The toxicity of AIDS drugs has been highly publicized in South Africa (Schneider & Fassin, 2002). AZT, one of the drugs used in PEP, has been singled out for toxic effects in the context of describing AIDS treatment as a Western plot to poison Africans (Schneider & Fassin, 2003). Messages about toxicity, many from figures in the ANC government, have stuck and require "reeducation." The OHS nurse at CH made reference to this:

> Some will say, "It is toxic, how can I take it?" But you say, no, like any medication it has side effects, it depends on the individual. Some go through it without any problem, others suffer. Of 28 reported, only 2 have refused PEP. (Zuma, OHS)

Zuma's explanation about drug toxicity was but one example of the professional and skillful manner in which she handled issues with the needlestick protocol. While 2 people completed PEP at DH, and 3 at RH, 26 completed the treatment at CH. Another factor that differed between the hospitals was the approach to side effects. Zuma described how she advised nurses who experienced nausea and headache to eat at particular times of the day: eat when taking the medication, and take the medication at night. In addition, she offered basic treatments for the symptoms. Having an OHS clinic to go to with these complaints, and a sympathetic staff to support them and remind them of the risk reduction supplied by the treatment, no doubt assisted nurses in completing the PEP regimen.

Few managers contemplated the overall problems suggested by the failure of the system for protecting nurses from occupational exposure to HIV. Although good in theory, nurses were not utilizing programs for reasons that were reasonably well understood. An exception was Dr. Holt at RH, and Zuma at CH. Holt felt that the state portrayed a lack of care for its staff through its programs; Zuma felt that support was the key element that management should provide.

> I think, overall, the state doesn't actively portray care for its staff. It doesn't go out of its way to say that the staff is as important as the patient. It's always Batho Pele principals, but no equivalent for the staff. Then there are rules for doctors and nurses, that you can't work at another institution. "No, no," everything is always negative. . . . The state could do a lot more to value the doctors and nurses. This definitely has an impact on patient care. Nurses only get 3,000 per month. So she will have to get another job just to have money to live. I don't know what the solution is, give incentives, raise salary. But many needs aren't monetary. Things like recognition, extra training, making ARV available. The state doesn't offer anything outside of the hospital that is confidential. Surely the state could offer a place for nurses and doctors. It is doing nothing, and that is frustrating. (Holt, MD)

> Health education is a process. It must be ongoing until it is seen that when it comes to HIV, management supports, so people feel that "I've got a shoulder to lean on." But if you find that the very same people you are working with are always negative, you will find you have no one. . . . As nurses, we need to have frequent workshops and opportunities to say, "Hey guys, we cannot conquer HIV/AIDS except to learn to be confident, to be an advocate, to say something if things are not done right as far as HIV is concerned. We need to be a supportive system. If we are always negative, what are we teaching? (Zuma, OHS)

Other Issues: Stress, HIV+ Staff

Hospital managers discussed issues associated with HIV+ nurses. Recently Dr. Nono Simelala, head of the National Department of Health's AIDS division, predicted that by 2015, 21% of nurses and 40% of nursing students would be HIV+ (Ncayiyana, 2004). While there are currently no reliable figures for HIV prevalence among nurses, one large community-based survey with a sound methodology predicted the HIV prevalence among nurses to be the same as that found in the general population (Shisana et al., 2004). At RH, the nurse manager did an informal review of absences and concluded that many appeared to be related to HIV/AIDS. CH reported three recent nurse deaths that they suspected to be HIV related, one confirmed.

Another problem for HIV infected nurses is exposure to TB. This is a problem because of the volume of TB patients and the increased presence of multidrug-resistant TB that requires longer, more complex treatment. TB-related mortality in AIDS patients is considerably higher than for TB patients without HIV infection.

> TB is a big issue now, we have MDRTB. They are increasing of late, due to HIV/AIDS. Before, not. But from the year 2000, we are having a lot of MDR. (Sizani, NM)

> Another huge problem is our HIV positive staff having to nurse patients with TB. But you have it throughout the hospital. TB is very common in our patients, there is no safe area, and HIV positive staff are at great risk nursing TB patients. From the OHS side, in the early days we attempted to isolate the problem. We tried to put HIV positive people in safe areas. But there are no more safe areas to put them, and there are so many staff affected. So the staff is just appointed as if no one is affected. (West, HM)

Hospital managers reported some problems with ARV treatment, including improper management by poorly trained private physicians and the high cost of treatment that must be covered out of pocket when Medical Aide is exhausted.

> Many Medical Aides pay for ARV. We have two doctors who are willing to see HIV positive patients and put them on treatment and monitor them. The problem is, HIV positive staff do take ARV, but they go to a private physician in town who doesn't necessarily know how the ARV should be administered. I've had feedback from the doctors that they are not administering them properly. I've written to the staff to let them know that the doctors are willing to see staff off premises, so they are assured of confidentiality. I've given out contact information and tried to encourage HIV positive staff to start on ARV and take care of themselves. But I believe only two have approached one of the doctors, and only one the other. People are just not willing to disclose their status. It isn't purely a problem with money, Medical Aide pays, the majority here pay for Medical Aide, so they are already paying! Other than GA and lower categories, the majority of nursing staff have Medical Aide. Dr. McNeill tried before I arrived, and I have tried since.

> There is another nurse, also positive, she came to me and disclosed her status, she said, "My problem is that I am sick frequently, I think I am going to be a nuisance in the wards. Maybe you can place me in a fully staffed ward so that my absence has less impact on the other staff." She is buying her own treatment, going to her laboratory—its R850 per month, and her Medical Aide has run out, she uses cash. The Medical Aide they take covers ARV, but they get exhausted quickly. Medical Aide has a cap, and it runs out. Its difficult to part with R850 per month. When she has children,

> other expenses, it becomes stressful. So most are moonlighting to supplement, people are resigning, going overseas, they want more money. (Zuma, OHS)

Hospital managers observed that nurses were exhausted and stressed out from working short of staff. The HR manager at CH noted that nurses worked much harder than other public-sector employees for the same pay, one reason he thought it was difficult to recruit them. The nursing manager at RH described how nurses are "exposed to short-staffing," and that this exposure caused stress and burn out. At DH, the nurse manager concluded that few nurses had problems with drugs or alcohol because they were "too tired from working short-staffed." The Hospital Manager at DH described that staff were stretched to an "unreasonable state."

CHAPTER SUMMARY

OHS programs cannot function in an environment where there is no open discussion of HIV/AIDS, and stigma and denial reign:

- Denial and stigma associated with HIV/AIDS led to failure to report needle-sticks, fear of VCT, and lack of discussion.
- Women's social position and government failures to respond exacerbated these problems for nurses.

The social context of the HIV/AIDS epidemic had severe consequences for OHS programs.

Impacts of social meaning of HIV/AIDS on OHS		
Denial		Underreporting
Stigma	→ →	Gossip
Women's position		Lack of open discussion
Government failure to respond		Only HIV negative report

- Nurses who did report and initiate PEP quit before the 1-month course was complete due to side effects.
- Some managers saw the problem of nurses' failure to report injuries and use precautions as an issue of compliance; others as a problem of support.

In addition to these road blocks to a successful OHS program to protect nurses from workplace exposures to HIV/AIDS, many of those who reported and initiated PEP to reduce their risk of sero-conversion quit due to side effects. Managers thought that they did not have sufficient knowledge of PEP. Some managers described the problems with OHS programs as a problem of nurses who were noncompliant and who refused to follow rules. Others viewed the problem in terms of insufficient support from the hospital and Department of Health for nurses' needs.

Staffing and OHS Programs in the Three Hospitals: Problems for Nurses are Not Affected Much by Whether the Hospitals are "Worlds Apart" or "World Class"

- Regardless of hospital setting, nurses migrated or moonlighted because of financial strains.
- And regardless of OHS setting, nurses failed to report blood exposures, avoided HIV tests, and didn't take PEP after an accidental blood exposure.

Assessing the situation for their nurses, managers concluded the following: Whether they worked in the beautiful world-class facility, the busy, overcrowded, regional hospital, or the remote, deprived rural hospital, nurses faced financial strains that pushed them to migrate overseas, leave retirement, or moonlight on top of full-time work. Whether they had access to a well-equipped occupational health clinic, good disposal bins, some needleless equipment, and reliable privacy measures or they lacked these things, nurses failed to report blood exposures, avoided the HIV test, and did not take PEP (despite the fact that it can reduce the chance of becoming HIV+ after an exposure by as much as 81%). Tables 5 and 6 summarize these conclusions.

Some managers—who viewed protecting nurses and implementing policy as part of their jobs—blamed nurses for noncompliance with OHS policy; others blamed the system for not providing adequate support. Both of these views represent a management perspective on this problem that does not consider the nurse's role in developing, evaluating, and implementing policy.

CHAPTER CONCLUSION

The brain drain of skilled health care workers from Africa to the developed world and the shortage of nurses that facilitates international migration played a

Table 5. Key Similarities in OHS and Nurse Staffing
at Three Hospitals

| Hospitals | Similarities | | | |
	Staff shortage characteristics	OHS utilization	Stress	Salaries
DH	• Low salaries primary reason for shortage	• Those who report are HIV negative	Stress and low morale	The same
RH	Overseas migration • Most severe deficit is professional nurses	• Underreporting Denial		
CH	• Rehiring retirees	Carelessness and negligence		

Table 6. Key Differences in OHS and Nurse Staffing
at Three Hospitals

| Hospitals | Differences | | | |
	Scale of staff shortages	Recruiting	OHS resources	Protocol implementation
DH	High % vacant, long time vacant, physician vacancies	No advantages, significant negatives include no entertainment, housing options.	No dedicated staff or space, good EAP, has H&S committee.	Few options for counseling. Poor resources for maintaining confidentiality.
RH	Increasing	Pleasant town, environment, good schools, good research opportunity.	Dedicated staff not trained in OHS, shares space, problems with EAP personnel, has H&S committee.	Few options for counseling. Poor resources for maintaining confidentiality.
CH	No current shortage at hospital	Outstanding environment, subsidized housing, strong recruitment program.	Dedicated trained staff and clinic EAP forming, highly structured H&S committee.	Good counseling options system and system for confidentiality.

significant role in the shortages in KZN hospitals. This situation is at odds with developing a labor-based approach to the HIV/AIDS epidemic because it weakens health systems and the base for developing power in the workforce. Given rising prices and new opportunities for South African nurses, the low salaries offered in the public sector are a significant problem.

Managers identified many ways in which OHS failed to protect nurses, despite the fact that the basics, such as systems for disposals, reporting needlestick injuries, workers compensation and post-exposure prophylaxis were available. Managers described how nurses did not utilize the policies available to them, and identified many reasons why this was the case. From an outsider's perspective, what is most strikingly lacking is nurses own participation in developing and implementing policies that could address the barriers to utilization.

The disparities between the hospitals also resulted in disparities in OHS programs across the provincial system, and again, the better supported and resourced facilities had advantages in terms of skills, equipment, and physical resources.

I now turn to the nurses' perspective on these issues.

CHAPTER 6

❦ ❧

Nurses Speak

We are short-staffed, trying to do too much, trying to get things done too
quickly. You rush, you are busy with the drip but you cannot concentrate, you
are rushing. (Medicine, RH)

Once you have the disease, it won't be seen as that you got the disease from
the patient, it won't be seen that I've got it from my husband, the whole
family, everyone, will think I was cheating. (Medicine, CH)

In this chapter, I present the views of 34 public-sector hospital nurses from the
three hospitals described in sections 1 and 2. I met with groups of 3 to 5 nurses at
the workplace on work time. In a scripted group interview setting they discussed
workplace blood exposures, hospital and government policy, and the impact of
HIV/AIDS on the workplace.

There are two limitations specific to the nurse group interviews that need to
be considered. First, nurses were recruited by management. This recruitment
method presents two problems: nurses may associate the interview with management or the Department of Health, or management may select nurses for a specific
reason. After going through the interview process, it appears that nurses were
selected based on convenience, and generally were simply summoned to come
to the appointed room with little explanation. Despite the introduction to the
project that was given to nurses, it is hard to appreciate what they thought about
it. In one case, a group of nurses approached me after the group interview to
ask about jobs in the United States, indicating that this may have been the
reason why they were interested in staying for the interview. At another meeting,
a nurse approached me to sort out a problem she was having with a union
benefit, so there may have been an assumption that I was connected to one of
the nurse's unions.

The other issue is the communication gap between a white American woman
who is not a nurse and South African, primarily Zulu, nurses. Overall, though the
perception may have been wrong, by the end of the majority of group interviews

it seemed that nurses were comfortable talking about their workplace issues. On the other hand, it is certain that many things were "lost in translation."

Overview

The conditions of work described in the previous chapters are the context for nurses' comments. These nurses work short-staffed, in some cases without crucial equipment, in an environment where management is struggling with resource issues. They work with many patients who are HIV positive and who also have TB. This includes many babies born to HIV positive mothers. The HIV status of patients is often not verified by a test, antiretroviral treatment for HIV/AIDS is not available, and family members are unaware of their loved ones' status. Despite the ubiquitous nature of HIV in the work environment, and frequent trainings, open discussion is lacking: the stigma of the disease carries over into the hospital, where nurses are hesitant to discuss it with patients. In this environment, confidentiality measures meant to protect nurses feed into secrecy and denial. Finally, nurses are struggling financially. They are paid lower than private-sector and international counterparts. This leads to out-migration to other countries or urban areas, moonlighting, and in some cases early retirement to get immediate access to benefit packages. Financial strains mean more short-staffing and overwork.

Despite the differences between the provincial hospitals in this study, hospital nurses' views are remarkably similar.[1] Hospital nurses reported that most accidental exposures to potentially hazardous blood occurred during injections and needle disposal, and were associated with rushing. Gloves were identified as the most important protection in such accidents, and nurses discussed the fact that gloves were frequently not worn at length. "Not wanting to know their own HIV status" was the main reason why nurses did not report blood exposures; and nurses did not take advantage of PEP in the event of exposures because they perceived that the drugs made you too sick and they did not want to be tested for HIV.

The nurses from the three provincial hospitals in this study observed that the HIV/AIDS epidemic had resulted in increases in the numbers of patients, and that these patients were sicker. Nurses described the HIV/AIDS epidemic as a major source of stress. They complained of overwork and poor conditions, and described being fearful of their own infection. At all hospitals, nurses described working short-staffed due to poor working conditions, and nurses seeking work abroad. Nurses described the process for reporting injuries as extensive and confusing. They felt that they were not recognized, underpaid, and blamed rather than supported when they were injured. And they identified the lack of ARV treatment as a significant problem.

Did the differences between the hospital settings influence hospital nurses' views on the impacts of HIV/AIDS, workplace exposures, and government and

---

[1] See Appendix for tables that compare views of nurses from each hospital.

hospital policies? While this study was not designed to discover associations between hospital characteristics and nurses' views, trends would have been evident from discussions among nurses prompted by the same questions. Though there were some differences between topics that emerged in group interviews, there was a striking degree of unanimity among nurses.[2] Due to the degree of similarities in responses from nurses, and the nature of the discussion in nine group interviews at three hospitals, there is then no reason to present the results from nurses by institution. One important caveat is that the nurses at the central hospital had been in their current jobs for a short time. Therefore, their opinions were mostly based on prior experiences at other hospitals. Since this hospital was on one end of the spectrum within the range of differences between hospitals, featuring the best working conditions, living conditions, and developed OHS program, it would be interesting to know whether or not, over time, nurses at CH would have different views. In the context of this study, and maximum hospital seniority of 1.5 to 2 years, they did not differ from their provincial counterparts.

Even given the short seniority at the central hospital, the fact that big differences in working conditions had little impact on nurses' views was striking. This seems to indicate that the factors that determine the work environment issues that are the same between hospitals—HIV/AIDS, low salaries, and nurses' lack of involvement in policymaking and implementation—are more important to nurses' OHS than the factors that make the settings distinct. And that even the best implemented policies and protocols are not adequate to address nurses' needs.

Workplace Exposure to HIV/AIDS

Many hospital nurses I interviewed did not view HIV/AIDS as an occupationally acquired disease.

> Most people think that it is mainly sexually transmitted. They think that chances of getting AIDS from the needle prick are very low. (Medicine, CH)

> I have only read about someone contracting the disease from a needle, I have never known of anyone who got it from a needle. (Maternity, DH)

This is not surprising: in 2001, 70% of the world's HIV-infected population lived in sub-Saharan Africa and only 4% of worldwide cases of occupational HIV infection were reported from this region (Sagoe-Moses et al., 2001). Prevention efforts focus primarily on sexual transmission. Hospital nurses indicated that HIV/AIDS is perceived primarily as a sexually transmitted, not occupationally acquired, disease, and that women were not in a position to demand safe sex even though they knew the risks.

[2]See Appendix.

> People don't believe in using condoms. He'll say no. (Medicine, RH)

> Husbands are coming from the mines with HIV, but women can't say wear a condom. (Medicine, DH)

Based on their understanding of HIV as sexually transmitted, hospital nurses linked the fear of becoming infected at work to fear of questions and gossip about their marital infidelity and sexual behavior. In the words of one professional-level hospital nurse from an adult medicine ward,

> Once you have the disease, it won't be seen as that you got the disease from the patient, it won't be seen that I've got it from my husband, the whole family, everyone, will think I was cheating. (Medicine, CH)

Nurses also expressed concern about their family's perceptions about their work with HIV/AIDS patients—that they would automatically contract the disease and, that if they were infected, their families would suffer disgrace. This contradicted the view that HIV/AIDS is not occupationally acquired, but underscored the stigma of working with HIV positive patients.

> They think that because I am here in the hospital, that I am going to contract AIDS. (AIDS Clinic, RH)

> If you are positive, the drugs won't work, and the whole world will know that you are positive. Your family, you will be humiliated and everyone will be talking about you. (Medicine, DH)

To summarize, nurses did not view workplace exposure to HIV/AIDS as a collective issue of workers rights and health on the job; rather, they discussed it in terms of stigma, women's disempowerment, and disgrace.

Universal Precautions, Gloves, and Protective Policies

Universal precautions were developed by the U.S. Center for Disease Control (CDC) in 1987 in response to the emergence of risk of HIV (and other bloodborne pathogens) to health care workers and others who provide care or first-aid (CDC, 1987). They state precautions should be used in the presence of all blood and body fluids.[3] Many nurses interviewed felt that aspects of universal precautions were unrealistic. Nurses complained that they couldn't wear gloves and other protective gear at all times, because of emergencies, being hurried, and lack of supplies.

---

[3] Including the use of personal protective equipment. The CDC guidelines, adopted by South Africa state: All health care workers should routinely use appropriate barrier precautions to prevent skin and mucous membrane exposure during contact with any patient's blood or body fluids that require universal precautions (CDC, 1987).

You can't be wearing gloves from morning until night. Not all patients are tested. It is what you are supposed to do, but it is not possible. (Maternity, CH)

You don't think of putting on gloves, you are in a hurry. (Medicine, RH)

There is gloves, mask, I have never seen them, only in the catalog. They are not issued. (Maternity, CH)

Supplies are out of stock, some sizes of gloves, and goggles are only provided for the doctors. I even said one day, I won't work if there is no goggles or mask. (Maternity, RH)

The use of gloves is a central component of universal precautions and is recommended for any contact with blood and body fluids, mucous membranes, or nonintact skin of all patients, for handling items or surfaces soiled with blood or body fluids, and for performing venipuncture and other vascular access procedures (Gerberding, 1995). Gloves have been shown to reduce the amount of blood involved in a needlestick exposure by 50% to 80%, depending on the type of device involved (Mast, Woolwine, & Gerberding, 1993). At the same time, gloves don't entirely prevent blood exposures, and nurses commented on this inadequacy.

Even if you wear the gloves, the needle still pokes through, so you will not be protected. (Medicine, DH)

The tone of some nurses' criticisms reflected the fact that that they believed those making the policies did not understand the situational context, and that the employer's main concern was to establish culpability should accidents occur.

I cannot come through the door and wear goggles and gloves until I go home at 6 pm. There is an emergency coming through the door. A splash gets into my eyes. Whatever the policies the government made, they never accommodated that part. Even when you are washing the patient, you are expected to wear goggles. I remember one colleague, she was washing a patient and she received a splash, before she was given an antiretroviral, she was asked for a statement to describe why she wasn't wearing the goggles. (Maternity, CH)

Universal precautions change the relationship between nurses and patients. A prime principal is that every patient contact be considered potentially risky. One nurse described feeling like a "ghost" or a "monster" instead of a human being when dealing with patients with protective gear on.

Coming from the patient's side, here comes the ghost wearing gloves and goggles, how do they feel? What are you saying to the patient, doing to the patient psychologically and socially? Now, every time we are going to touch the patient, we wear goggles and gloves? We look like a monster. These things must be taken into account. (Medicine, RH)

> Our mothers say that we used to touch the patients. We used to wash them, we used to catch the baby bare hands. Now the patient doesn't understand that we can't catch the baby with our bare hands. They think that you are cruel. (Maternity, RH)

Nurses noted that despite the edict to "treat all patients as positive," it wasn't really possible.

> You are supposed to treat each and every patient as if they are positive. Take the same precautions. But if you know they are (HIV) positive, it is not the same as treating the negative patient. (Medicine, DH)

This simple statement captures the sense in which to "treat all alike" is absurd; nurses know that it feels different to care for patients they know to be HIV positive.

How Do Accidental Exposures Occur?

Hospital nurses described specific situations that most frequently resulted in needlesticks.

> Suturing in the labor ward, you are holding the patient, not using an instrument, you are using one hand to steady the hemorrhage. The patient is moving about, most do not stay still. (Maternity, DH)[4]

> Restless, confused patients. You must hold the patient with one hand, and the needle is already in one hand. (Medicine, RH)

> If you are not concentrating when removing the needle. It is mostly a prick from the right hand into the left hand. Somehow you lose concentration after giving the injection. (Medicine, CH)

> From where I come from. People do not take necessary precautions. I don't know if it is carelessness or what, but they are pricked. As you say, patients aren't screened. (Maternity, CH)

> I don't know if nurses are careless. But you are not supposed to dislodge the needle, you have to put in the sharps container without dislodging, but some try to dislodge it. They are not sure if patient is positive or not. (AIDS Clinic, RH)

---

[4] For the U.S. reader, it is important to note the difference in the tasks that maternity nurses perform compared to U.S. nurses and the impact on exposure risk. Suturing a patient, who is not necessarily anesthetized, is not done by nurses in the United States and presents a strong potential exposure to blood/sharps exposure, though with a lower risk (not hollow bore) needle.

Nurses attribute accidents to patient movement, nurse's carelessness, improper disposal, and a loss of concentration while performing procedures. Loss of concentration and not thinking were related to rushing and short-staffing.

> We are short-staffed, trying to do too much, trying to get things done too quickly. You rush, you are busy with the drip but you cannot concentrate, you are rushing. (Medicine, RH)

> You don't think of putting on gloves, you are in a hurry. (Maternity, DH)

Hospital nurses also described accidents as inherent to the nature of their work in emergency situations.

> When we are rushing a bleeding patient to surgery. In those cases we are saving a life, as we are risking ours. There is no other way we could have done that. (Medicine, CH)

> In emergency situations, in many situations you do not think of your own safety, you think of the patient first. (Medicine, RH)

Reporting and Forms

When a needlestick injury is reported, nurses must fill out an injury-on-duty form. Nurse's described the forms as humiliating, annoying, and the process as long.

> If you prick yourself, you must report . . . you must record "How did you poke yourself?" That writing, it is humiliating. As if you were too careless to poke yourself. (Medicine, CH)

> But we know that there is a procedure to follow. But sometimes you find that people are afraid. It is a long procedure. We have to do this for safety. But it is too long. (Medicine, DH)

> Some report and some don't. The way of answering that form, it is annoying, as if you took a needle and you poked yourself. They want to know how did you poke yourself. There is a spot from the needle, it went in. How did it happen, I don't know? But I ended poked. But they will tell me to write it down. At the end of the day, I am not going there. (Maternity, RH)

In particular, nurses believed they were treated as careless when accidents occurred.

> The people who are at the head of the department, they don't accept that you have been extra careful. As if you like to be poked. (Medicine, CH)

Some nurses suggested that someone should be available to help them fill out forms properly in the midst of the stress and worry of a potentially hazardous accident.

> I don't think the forms need to be changed, but you should be given a guide. Money won't be paid if it is your carelessness. (AIDS Clinic, RH)

> Someone should help you, to tell you what to write. She is already a patient, she is stressed, she needs help. What about me, what about my family, what about my husband, what will happen? I will lose my whole family, what am I going to tell them, and at the end of the day, the employer is humiliating you . . . how did you get it? (Maternity, DH)

This last quote captures the sense, expressed by many nurses, that the employer/government seemed not to appreciate that a workplace blood exposure was a great cause of personal worry and stress. For nurses, the employer appeared concerned only with liability.

Reporting and Voluntary Counseling and Testing (VCT)

Hospital protocol following accidental exposure to blood required that a health worker be tested for HIV after reporting the incident and taking a stat dose of PEP. Fear of a test result that shows a nurse is already HIV+ at the time of an accidental exposure was identified as the primary deterrent to the HIV test.

> I think the main thing is that you are scared to take the blood to be checked. At the same time, if the results come back positive, people are scared of the result. (AIDS Clinic, DH)

> Drugs depend on the results (of the HIV test). If you are positive, the drugs won't work, and the whole world will know that you are positive. Your family, you will be humiliated and everyone will be talking about you. (Medicine, CH)

> Others are afraid. What if I report and the results say that I am positive and the patient is negative? (Maternity, DH)

Nurses characterized this fear by reference to sudden, life-changing knowledge:

> People are afraid to have the blood test. This happened to my friend. They drew her blood, and the test came back positive. Just imagine yourself, just coming to work in the morning, not knowing anything, and all of a sudden. That will affect your whole life. So that is why people are afraid to check the blood, and to report the incident. I think there are three times more sticks than what is reported. (Medicine, RH)

In the following exchange, nurses discuss the fact that patients are not required to be tested for HIV, though they are. They questioned why the test was necessary for PEP, and suggested that changing the policy that requires nurses to be tested could increase reporting.[5] While changing the policy is problematic, this exchange precisely reveals nurses' issues with this policy: patients' rights are valued over nurses' rights, and nurses do not want to know their HIV status.

> Patients are not forced to give blood. So why must I? If I don't want to give blood, they must just give me the ARV. (Medicine, RH)

> The policy must change, so that if you get a needlestick, you get treatment. But you don't have to have blood taken. (Medicine, RH)

> Logically they will never report it . . . just ignore it . . . the policy is just made in a way, I don't know who it favors. They ask you to take blood. (Medicine, RH)

> More people would report if this policy was changed. (Medicine, RH)

As a group, hospital nurses seemed to accept the logic that it was better not to know your HIV status if there was no treatment available, as reflected in this comment:

> If they are going to be treated for HIV, then it makes sense to report, otherwise it won't help. (Medicine, CH)

Hospital nurses were nearly unanimous in the opinion that the lack of access to affordable ARV treatment contributed to the reluctance to be tested. In May 2003 the policy that will make ARV treatment available in public hospitals had not yet been approved.[6] Many hospital nurses indicated a distrust of hospital measures to ensure the confidentiality of their test result, though provincial DoH policy requires that each health worker tested be given a number and HIV test results kept confidential. The size of hospitals and close proximity of staff were reasons given for distrust of confidentiality measures.

Post-Exposure Prophylaxis (PEP)

Post-exposure prophylaxis has been available in South Africa through the public sector since 2001 (KZN, 2001). However, most hospital nurses I interviewed who volunteered that they had used PEP said that they did not complete the treatment because of side effects. Many who had not taken the drugs repeated

---

[5] This suggestion is problematic, because even small exposures to ARVs can lead to resistance. An HIV positive person using PEP could reduce the effectiveness of future ARV treatment for HIV. This could be an important issue as treatment becomes available to more people.

[6] Though approved, this policy has not been fully implemented. Only 10 sites are certified to offer ARV in KZN as of 2005.

stories about friends who had, and agreed that PEP drugs could not be tolerated. Many thought that the government only looked at the price of PEP drug regimens and not the side effects. Although PEP has been associated with as much as an 81% reduction of risk for HIV sero-conversion after percutaneous exposure to HIV-infected blood (Gerberding, 2003), adverse side effects to PEP drugs were discussed by study participants to a great extent, while the potential risk reduction associated with PEP was not. In this exchange, that was characteristic of the discussion of PEP in group interviews, three nurses talked about the side effects of PEP drugs.

> Another reason that people don't report is that people say the antiretroviral drugs make them sick. (Medicine, CH)
>
> Once you report and give blood, you have to go on the drugs. (Medicine, CH)
>
> They make you sick (everyone agrees)! (Medicine, CH)
>
> It makes you nauseous all the time, constipated. (Medicine, CH)
>
> I've taken it, and I stopped. (Medicine, CH)
>
> I also took it for 2 weeks only. The treatment is horrible. They cause amnesia, you have an itchy body, you don't sleep at night, you don't eat, you feel miserable. (Medicine, CH)
>
> I took it for 2 or 3 weeks, and I was so sick I couldn't work. Why didn't the doctors tell me? I'd rather die of AIDS than die of treatment. (Medicine, CH)

This conversation was replicated in most interviews when the subject of PEP was raised. It is notable that all agreed about the side effects, whether they had taken the drugs or not. The perception that reporting meant that you must take the drugs presents the possibility that avoiding PEP was actually a reason to not report. While this makes little sense in terms of nurses' knowledge of transmission, the ravages of the disease, and the potential of PEP to prevent infection, it does make sense in terms of the view that the hospital is forcing PEP upon nurses, that it is for liability protection rather than protecting nurses.

The distrust of the PEP program is reflected in the following exchange about the choice of PEP drugs.

> The government policy supplies only AZT and 3TC. I know someone else who got the treatment through Medical Aide, and they were ordered some treatment, and they were not sick. I think what is happening is that we are taking drugs also, but we are only keeping one drug (regimen), it cannot be changed. There are some better antiretroviral drugs, but they are very expensive. (Medicine, CH)
>
> Yes, these other drugs are too expensive, so the government decided to bring this AZT which is much cheaper. And we don't take this treatment, and we are dying. (Medicine, CH)

So why don't they change the drugs? Maybe it is because we don't go back and tell the doctor. (Medicine, CH)

This reflects the suspicion that, for financial reasons, public-sector nurses are denied treatments with fewer side effects. Nurses see the quality of PEP as another reflection of underresourcing of their work environment and lack of concern for nurses by the government (as distinguished from the hospital). Criticisms of AZT are complicated by the fact that the toxicity of AZT in particular has been a big topic in the media because of the government controversy over HIV/AIDS (Schneider & Fassin, 2002). At the end of this exchange, one nurse hints at the fact that nurses quit the drugs but don't inform the doctor, pointing to a missed opportunity to raise the problems from the nurse perspective.

The bottom line for nurses and PEP is that even if they go through the process up to the point of getting PEP—the injury is reported, nurses consent to a test, their test is negative—many do not complete the course of treatment.

I've never met one person who told me, "I took ARV for the whole course." No one. (Medicine, DH)

This isn't surprising, given that one third of U.S. health workers on the PEP registry discontinued treatment because of side effects (Gerberding, 2003).

I have a colleague who took the treatment, and he is positive anyway. It doesn't work all the time. (AIDS Clinic, RH)

Impacts of HIV/AIDS

Physical and psychosocial stress was the major impact of the HIV/AIDS epidemic on the nurses' role as described by hospital nurses. Workload increases attributed to increased patient census and acuity, and staff shortages—particularly of the more skilled nurses—were identified as contributing to the physical and psychosocial demands of the job. Hospital nurses described HIV-related changes to the nurse/patient relationship that they found stressful.

Increases in HIV/AIDS and TB Patients

Nurses described the impacts of the HIV/AIDS epidemic on their workplaces, specific jobs, and lives. The numbers of HIV/AIDS and TB patients are increasing and problems such as teen pregnancy are exacerbated.

I have been concerned. The number of HIV positive patients is increasing, more and more are positive. Most are TB positive. You are scared that you can catch the TB. (AIDS Clinic, DH)

Seventy-five percent are positive that we see, and it is increasing daily. People don't believe in using condoms. (Medicine, RH)

We used to just have a problem of teenage pregnancies. Now they are getting pregnant, and getting AIDS. After all this, you would think teenage pregnancy rate would decrease. The rate is still the same, as if they don't know anything about AIDS. But they do. They know the signs and the symptoms, they can tell you, "that one is suffering, this one is suffering." (Maternity, DH)

Infected Coworkers

Nurses' experiences of HIV positive coworkers were not positive, even if the exposure had an occupational source. Coworkers did not support each other.

There was one chap at King Edward, a professional nurse, he had a human bite from a patient, at the end of the day he was positive, and the whole hospital knew. He was infected, people were not supportive, they humiliated him. (Medicine, CH)

Nurses described how the HIV status of coworkers was the subject of gossip, not concern and support.

Nurse/Patient Relationship

HIV/AIDS brought about changes in the maternity nurse/patient relationship. The celebration and excitement around the birth of a child that came with the job of being a maternity nurse disappeared; expectant mothers sick with AIDS avoided prenatal care; and the human intimacy between patient and nurse is disturbed by the risk of infection.

You are nursing patients, most are positive, you have to be extra careful. Patients come in with so many problems, and also psychological problems. The patient is weak, sick, stressed, it all has to be attended to. When a woman came to give birth, it used to be a celebration. Now if the mother is very sick, there is little excitement. Some are very very sick. (Maternity, RH)

They don't even come until they are about to give birth. Then they expect us to rush to give birth to that baby. We say "nonclinic mothers" because they have not had prenatal care. (Maternity, RH)

They should come 2 to 3 months ahead, but now they just stay in there house until they are ready to deliver. They don't want to be talked about. (Maternity, RH)

They don't even listen; they don't know what to do giving birth. (Maternity, RH)

Our mothers say that we used to touch the patients. We used to wash them; we used to catch the baby with bare hands. Now the patient doesn't understand that we can't catch the baby with our bare hands. They think that you are cruel. (Maternity, RH)

Maintaining the confidentiality of a patient's HIV status made nurses uncomfortable, and is another way that HIV/AIDS has changed the nurse/patient relationship. Confidentiality is part of a number of workplace HIV/AIDS policies;[7] in South Africa spouses are supposed to be notified of patients' status. Nurses were quite uncomfortable with coming between family members.

We are supposed to hide everything. A family wanted to come into theater while the mother was giving birth, they wanted to know if the baby would be given prophylaxis. The mother-in-law was pressuring us. But the mother did not want to reveal her status. This was very stressful. (Maternity, CH)

Nurses as HIV Educators

Some nurses had anxiety about answering a patient's questions related to treatment for HIV/AIDS. They felt undereducated.

I don't think that there is anyone who is clear about HIV, who really knows. I think we are just all trying to put the facts together. (Medicine, CH)

The use of the ARV niviripine for PMTCT has been a policy in KZN since 2002 (Willan, 2004), after a struggle between provincial and national departments of health.[8] Maternity nurses' comments revealed that they were not equipped to answer basic, logical questions about PMTCT.

If the ARV works for the baby, why not the mother?[9] (Maternity, RH)

I find myself in a debate, because people ask a lot of questions. How is it possible that mother is positive and baby negative, when baby gets the blood from the mother?[10] So you find yourself confused too. (Maternity, RH)

Lack of information made patient education on HIV stressful for nurses and impeded open discussion.

[7] See previous chapter description of confidentiality policies.

[8] In 2002, two provinces, Guateng and KZN, made a decision to begin a PMTCT program despite the fact that national government had opposed the decision.

[9] Prevention of mother to child transmission (PMTCT) involves a single dose of neviripine administered to mother and baby during childbirth. It is intended to prevent transmission from mother to child, not to treat HIV/AIDS in the mother.

[10] This topic reveals misinformation about the blood supply of the fetus in utero. Risk of infection from mother to child is during the birth process.

Community/Hospital Linkages

Nurses experienced the HIV/AIDS epidemic at home and at work, but felt that this wasn't discussed.

> I am coming from a place where a lot of people are dying from AIDS. (AIDS Clinic, DH)

> Our brothers and sisters come to the hospital, and they see the people dying of HIV/AIDS, and who is nursing them? It is us, their brothers and sisters, so they know, but hey, this is so and so, nobody wants to discuss this. (AIDS Clinic, RH)

> The hospital sends people home when they are very sick, but people don't know how to care for them. We see this in the community. (AIDS Clinic, RH)

Nurses described feeling stressed, afraid, and miserable because of their multiple daily exposures to HIV/AIDS and its impacts.

> This disease also affects our social lives. We work with this everyday, and we read the stories in the paper. We become more afraid, we find ourselves sitting at home. It makes our life miserable. (Medicine, CH)

Nurses described the need for more community education on HIV in light of the fact that what happens in the community makes a difference for what happens in the hospital.

> Many husbands are coming from the mines with HIV, but women can't say wear a condom. The issues in the community make a difference to what happens in the hospital. We need more people to teach the community. So many people are ignorant. (AIDS Clinic, RH)

Workplace and Government Policy

During the scripted group interviews, I asked nurses to evaluate government policy on HIV/AIDS and workplace exposure to HIV in relation to their jobs. The discussions that ensued were characterized by two interrelated themes: the undervaluing of hospital nurses and lack of government commitment to fighting the HIV/AIDS epidemic.

> I don't think government or Department of Health does enough for us or the patients, though the hospital might wish to. (Medicine, RH)

Workers Compensation

Lack of compensation for workplace injury and risk reflected how nurses are undervalued.

I think you are supposed to get some compensation from the government. There are some procedures to follow from your injury. But they have strong rules—that is why it is humiliating. You will not receive the compensation, and you will be humiliated. (Maternity, RH)

Hospital and department of health do not do enough to compensate workers for risks. They don't give compensation. They blame carelessness. (Medicine, RH)

Others such as firefighters and those in the military are compensated for risks. We aren't recognized. (Medicine, RH)

Salaries and "Going Overseas"

One of the chief ways that nurses expressed feeling undervalued was salaries. I did not ask specifically about salaries in the scripted interviews, but at the end of each group session I asked if there was anything I had missed that they thought was important for me to know. Invariably, nurses said that they were underpaid and struggling.

We do not earn enough. Salaries are too low to survive. (Medicine, DH)

This pay is only enough if you are living in a shack, not if you want something better. (Medicine, CH)

The price of food and everything has gone up, but salaries have not. Even after many years, we will not earn enough. (Maternity, RH)

The solution for many nurses was to seek work overseas.[11] However, leaving for higher paying jobs came at great cost and sacrifice to nurses and their families.

Many go for a year to earn enough to pay their mortgage, and then they come back. Relatives care for their children while they are gone. (Maternity, CH)

The ones who go to Saudi Arabia have a terrible time. The culture is very different, and they don't expect it when they go. (Medicine, CH)

One nurse who went to Britain lived in a place where she was the only black. Everyone stared at her. They expect it to be better than it is. There, it is expensive and hard to save. Our nurses who go get the worst jobs. (Medicine, CH)

---

[11] Nurses informed me about a recruiter located in Durban that many nurses were working with to secure arrangements and paperwork for contracts in Britain and Saudi Arabia. Many were making contact via the Internet or phone.

Nurses who leave for overseas sacrifice everything—their families, children, husbands, and homes—but they must go because they need the money. (Maternity, DH)

HIV/AIDS Policy

Nurses discussed how government's messages about the causes of HIV/AIDS undercut prevention and behavior change efforts.

When someone who people believe, like the president, tells people that AIDS isn't the killer, that it is all about starvation, this is a serious problem. People think, "Why should I wear a condom?" (Medicine, CH)

Finally, nurses abhorred government's neglect of AIDS treatment[12] and its role in sending confusing messages about the disease.[13]

Our government here, they tell you that AIDS is caused by poverty. So we definitely know that these people don't care. (AIDS Clinic, RH)

The government says, "We can't do anything for you," there are no drugs to be given to the patient. (Medicine, DH)

Occupational Health Policy

Nurses' specific criticisms of occupational health policy touched on inadequate confidentiality, lack of treatment for nurses, dissatisfaction with forms and processes that are humiliating and annoying, PEP drug side effects, and the fact that an HIV test is required for PEP; this has been the major topic of this section. Overall, nurses described how workplace-exposure policy seemed to benefit the hospital not the nurses. Some nurses suggested that policies be restructured.

People are not protected. They must go back and restructure the policies. (AIDS Clinic, RH)

The lowest classes of workers are not protected. The policies are written in English. The GA[14] doesn't know English. She is working with a mop. There are needles down there. You tell her to wear the gloves, but she doesn't see why. They are uncomfortable. They need to restructure and help people. And change the treatment; offer different treatment and don't think about finances all the time. (Medicine, RH)

Nurses' suggestions for safer work are summarized in Box 1.

---

[12] See Chapter 4 for a history of government actions on HIV/AIDS treatment policy.

[13] Key ANC figures have spread the message that AIDS is not caused by HIV, and that ARV drugs are toxic. See Willan (2004) and Schneider (2002).

[14] General Assistant.

Box 1: Nurses' recommendations for safer work

How can injury reports and PEP uptake be increased?
- Provide ARV treatment to nurses and other health care workers
- Switch to PEP drug regimens with more favorable side effects
- Assistance with incident reports and compensation forms at the time of injury
- Additional training about PEP and risk
- Reduce humiliation of reporting

How can injuries be prevented?
- Increase staffing
- Provide appropriate protective equipment (gloves, goggles, masks)
- Staff development and education
- Written policies in all languages, special training for general assistants

How can nurse interactions with HIV positive patients be improved?
- Community education about HIV/AIDS
- Open discussion
- Consider people first, not finances

Notes on Interpreting Contradictions

During these interviews, nurses made statements that appear to be contradictory. Examples of contradictions include the following:

- Nurses say that they should be able to get PEP automatically after a needlestick without being tested, but that they don't want PEP and it doesn't work anyway.
- Nurses say that gloves and goggles aren't available, but (in the same facility) also say that they're pressured to wear them all the time when they don't want to.
- Nurses say that everyone believes that HIV is only sexually transmitted, not occupationally transmitted, but others report that family members expect them to get the infection from working at the hospital.

I reported what appeared to be the predominant themes based on these interviews, but there were of course variations among individuals. The first two examples here show a specific trend. Nurses were critical of hospitals policies and their commitment to their own policies. Thus, they dislike the PEP they are offered and the physical protections, but they also state that these things aren't readily available.

Three Additional Noteworthy Discussions

Three exchanges occurred that are noteworthy but didn't fit neatly into categories. Only the first was part of a recorded, formal group interview.

During a group interview among maternity nurses at the regional hospital, nurses expressed a strong desire for openness through a discussion that was prompted by this comment.

> I am so tired of secrecy. We should have a hospital for HIV/AIDS, where the nurses are also HIV positive. Then no one will have to hide. We will not have this confidentiality, and we can discuss openly. (Maternity, RH)

Other nurses strongly agreed with this statement, and there was a feeling of empowerment in the room that came with this suggestion. With more discussion, nurses would have likely arrived at the downside to this suggestion, but the desire for open discussion was palpable.

In an informal meeting of older Indian nurses—most retired or in management at R. K. Kahn hospital—nurses discussed how Muslims, Christians, and Hindus from the Indian communities had struggled with addressing issues of sexuality in the context of facing HIV/AIDS. They explained that there was a strong edict in the Indian communities that said that "these things are not a problem for us." This issue did not come up in group interviews with nurses, but clearly would be an issue for all nurses, given the conservativeness of African communities as well.

Another discussion in an informal meeting with unionized nurses from three nurse's unions held at McCord's hospital focused on the question of who confidentiality benefits. This group saw stigma as benefiting a government that didn't want to deal with the problem of HIV/AIDS. They felt that the government actually cultivated stigma and denial in their approach to HIV/AIDS in order to maintain power and avoid the costs of treating the disease and attending to other public health problems. In their view, as long as people were silenced by stigma and denial, it is unlikely that they will stand together openly and demand health, workplace, and human rights.

As if They Liked to be Poked, Migrate Overseas, and Remain Silenced!

Overall, nurses' views corroborated managers' descriptions of how denial, stigma, women's position, and government failures led to problems with implementing OHS measures. However, their perspective expands and characterizes how policies fail. They found the process of reporting injuries humiliating, and nurses felt that policies protected patient's rights but not nurses. They felt the government and department of health were more concerned with liability than nurse protection, and that the stress of the experience of the needlestick ("I will lose my whole family") wasn't appreciated by those who made the policies. Finally, nurses thought that the implication of their carelessness in sharps injuries showed that the government did not appreciate that the job of the nurse, in the context of emergencies and close patient contact, was inherently risky ("you think of the patient, not your own safety").

- Nurses did not trust that government policy was meant to protect them.
  Nurses' distrust of government was revealed in their distrust of PEP. They were very quick to believe that better PEP drugs were denied them due to government's indifference to side effects. In some sense, this is probably true; it is common for public health dictates to weigh risks and benefits in such a way that minimizes individual discomforts/downsides.
- Nurses migrate for overseas jobs because of low salaries.
- Short-staffing due to shortage contributes to injuries.
- Migration means huge sacrifices for the nurse and her family.

Nurses trace short-staffing to overseas migration, and therefore to financial strain brought on by low salaries. Rushing and poor concentration while handling too many patients provides a link between short-staffing and sharps injuries. Nurses described the sacrifices that nurses made in order to work overseas: far from being the easy choice to earn more money, going to Saudi Arabia or Britain for work meant leaving family and community, and suffering discrimination. As nurses explained, the public sector salary was fine if you lived in a shack, revealing that third world living conditions were part of the calculus upon which these salaries were based.

- HIV/AIDS has dramatically altered the nurse/patient relationship and the content of the nursing job.
  Nurses described how the nurse/patient relationship was disrupted by HIV/AIDS. The change in the quality of the jobs of maternity nurses was clear in these interviews: jobs that had once included the benefit of being a part of a joyful experience were now marked by the problems of nonclinic mothers and the tragedy of illness. Nurses who once felt close to the patients they nursed now felt like monsters.

- Nurses blamed ANC-led government for failing to address HIV/AIDS.
  Nurses were very critical of the ANC-led government's HIV/AIDS policy, especially claims that AIDS was caused by poor nutrition and poverty and the failure to provide ARV treatment. This was part of the overall sense that nurses, on the frontlines of an infectious disease epidemic, were unrecognized, undervalued, and unprotected. Despite a lack of openness about HIV/AIDS, and admittance that their attitudes engendered stigma and denial, nurses expressed a strong desire for openness and change.

- Nurses' views were the same across settings that differed greatly in terms of physical resources and OHS programs, indicating that
  - The factors that determine the work-environment issues that are the same between hospitals—HIV/AIDS, low salaries, and nurses' lack of involvement in policymaking and implementation—are more important to nurses' OHS than the factors that make the settings distinct.
  - Policies and protocols are not adequate to address nurses' needs.

The lack of variation of nurses' views despite differences in settings and resources suggests that whatever investments result in these differences do not affect the problems nurses face. Nurses' financial struggles due to low salaries, exacerbated by high prices and high unemployment, link their individual situations to wider economic conditions in which inequality is high and the working class struggle. Stigma, denial, and lack of antiretroviral treatment were consequences of the Mbeki-led ANC government's failure to address HIV/AIDS, and were the key factors that impeded how OHS programs were utilized. At the same time, the fact that nurses and their unions were only minimally involved with OHS programs at the hospital level was striking. This was a fact notable by omission, not something that nurses commented on except to say, "We don't know who these policies are meant to benefit."

CHAPTER CONCLUSION

Nurses described feeling undervalued for their work in terms of pay, recognition, and the attitudes of the Department of Health toward HIV/AIDS and nurses' role. Opinions about OHS reflected these attitudes. Nurses viewed policies and protocols as geared toward protecting the employer in terms of liability and blaming nurses for accidental injuries. This suspicion was fed by ongoing misinformation from the government about HIV/AIDS and treatment, and their own experience of the results of policy failures—increasing numbers of HIV/AIDS and TB patients.

Social issues, especially gender issues, were important. This suggests that developing a labor-based approach to HIV/AIDS involving nurses would need to specifically address gender issues within and outside of the workplace.

Next, I turn to a discussion of this case study in the context of the background of neoliberalism and its impacts on health policy in South Africa and recommendations for a labor/work-environment approach to HIV/AIDS that follow.

CHAPTER 7

ભ ૪૦

Discussion

Breathing Life into Policy:
Toward a Labor/Work Environment
Perspective on a Global Public Health Crisis

Despite the postapartheid health system development program of district-based
PHC developed through the legacy of the progressive public health movement
in South Africa and enshrined in principle in the 1995 White Paper on the
transformation of the Health system, and a specific policy of shifting from curative
to preventative care, this study of three provincial hospitals found disparities
between them that favored the more specialized hospitals. These disparities also
correlated with neoliberal health policy principles: the private/public partnership
that shifts public health spending to the private sector and efforts to recoup
Medical Aide funds in the private sector led to dynamism and system support in
the better resourced settings.

However, contrary to what might be anticipated, these differences in setting
didn't matter for the occupational health issues of nurses. Despite a huge variation
in occupational health services (OHS), nurses described the same problems:
stigma around HIV/AIDS; many reasons not to report exposures (which led to
underreporting, failure to be tested or to take post-exposure prophylaxis [PEP]);
and the feeling that they were not supported, protected, or appreciated at the
highest levels of management. Further, nurses at all three hospitals described
OHS programs and policies that they were not part of developing or implementing.
Nurses discussed occupational health and safety and HIV/AIDS in terms of
stigma, denial, and disgrace—not workplace rights.

Specifically, the hospital case studies based on manager and nurse interviews
reveal the following:

- There was a wide range of difference between the physical settings of the
  three hospitals: from "world class" to "third world."
- There were enormous disparities in resources and staff between the three
  hospitals; and this disparity was reflected in OHS programs.

- Denial and stigma associated with HIV/AIDS led to failure to report needle-sticks, fear of VCT, and lack of discussion; this was exacerbated by women's social position and government's failure to respond to HIV/AIDS.
- Low salaries are the primary cause of overseas migration for nursing jobs that has led to a shortage of nurses. Financial problems also push nurses to moonlight, and retirees back into hospital employment.

Despite disparities between the hospitals, and the community health implications, similarities were more important than differences for nurses' occupational health:

- Regardless of OHS setting, nurses failed to report blood exposures, avoided HIV tests, and didn't take PEP after an accidental blood exposure.
- The factors that determine the work environment issues that are the same between hospitals—HIV/AIDS, low salaries, and nurses' lack of involvement in policymaking and implementation—are more important to nurses' OHS than the factors that make the settings distinct.
- Policies and protocols are not adequate to address nurses' needs.

The health system investments, and their unequal division between hospitals, don't seem to accrue much benefit for key aspects of nurses work experiences.

Key Background Points Revisited

In the preceding chapters I developed a rich context for the occupational health and safety issues faced by South African public-sector hospital nurses, which is important in understanding the dilemmas that nurses face and the scope and content of solutions to these dilemmas. The public sector hospital work environment in South Africa has been determined by the legacy of colonialism and apartheid rule, and by structural adjustment programs (SAPS) in the 1980s and the international ascendance of neoliberal globalization in the years that followed. This has had a profound influence on the physical and financial resources of the public health system in South Africa and on the provincial and national health policies that shape the system. As a basis for the discussion that follows about the implications of this study for a labor/work-environment approach to a global public health crisis, it is useful to revisit the key points of this background.

In the 1980s the debt crisis and SAPs marked the end of a brief period of the social and economic national development of newly independent African countries. The SAPs meant the loss of national sovereignty over policy—including health policy—and specific restrictions on public investments in health. These changes not only led to increased poverty and decreased access to health services, but also to a reversal of public health policy based on the Primary Health Care (PHC) model exemplified by the 1978 Alma Ata declaration. This was not only the abandonment of a functional model, but of a thorough analysis of what type of health system could address the political, economic, and social dimensions of health, as well as the sickness and care of individuals (Loewenson, 1993; Turshen, 1999). In particular, the PHC model was replaced by "selective strategies," which reduced PHC to an approach to addressing particular health issues (Banerji, 1999). This approach narrowed the scope of health issues, reduced the number and type of things that governments would be responsible for, and provided a model more amenable to privatization. Important health indicators in sub-Saharan African countries declined in this period; for example, Zimbabwe experienced near halving of infant mortality rates after it began a public PHC program following independence in 1980. After instituting its SAP, the central hospital in Harare recorded an 88% increase in maternal deaths between 1989 and 1990, and a 22% increase in the number of infant deaths between 1990 and 1991 (Turshen, 1999). Naturally, these disinvestments in public health played out in the deteriorating conditions of work for nurses and other health care workers.

South Africa won democracy/independence after years of popular struggle and held its' first election in 1994. The newly elected African National Congress (ANC) had been the lead organization of the antiapartheid liberation movement, but the ANC was quickly hamstrung by the worldwide trends toward neoliberal policies. Despite years of struggle for the economic and social rights of poor black South Africans, the new government replaced the social development framework that had been the guiding document for transformation from apartheid to democracy with market-oriented macroeconomic policy (Bond, 2004a). South Africa had a rich legacy of progressive health policy that laid the groundwork for health policy in the era of democracy. For example, the 1997 plan for health sector development outlined a district-based primary health care system that included the means of harnessing benefits from the private sector (RSA, 1997). The 1990 Maputo Statement laid out an approach to addressing HIV/AIDS that took into account the social, economic, and political dimensions of the disease (Stein & Zwi, 1990). But the 1996 shift in macroeconomic policy constrained these efforts by limiting investments, increasing poverty and inequality, and decisively orienting the policy environment toward neoliberal values that claimed that economic adjustments could lead development efforts. The human development index (HDI), a composite figure that reflects health and development data, fell below it's apartheid-era score in 2001 after peaking in 1995 (United Nations Development Programme [UNDP], 2004). Between 1996 and 2000, South Africa lost 400,000 jobs each year (Congress of South African Trade Unions [COSATU], 2000). The HIV/AIDS epidemic exploded in South Africa during the same period, offering the starkest example of disturbing trends.

In KwaZulu-Natal, public hospital system development since 1994 has reflected two trends. The first, in line with the goals of expanding access to care and care quality in the public sector, has been to combine formerly segregated services and to add new services (such as clinics to facilitate the district based, primary preventative care model, and the new central hospital for tertiary/quaternary services). The second has been to introduce privatization measures into the public sector, primarily as a way to improve quality or increase revenue. Specific examples from this study are the private/public partnership (PPP) at the central hospital, and the devotion of medical facilities to private-pay patients at the regional hospital. While these measures do not necessarily contradict the development of the district-based PHC system, it is alarming that the district hospital in the study suffered continued neglect and that the PPP model has received such extensive support and attention. This is evidence that the priorities of the Health Department have been skewed by the focus on the financial side.

The international labor situation for nursing is shaped by neoliberalism and has been problematic for nurses and health systems worldwide. Within the framework of the international increase in commodification and privatization of health services (Navarro, 2004), the "global nursing shortage" has been driven in large part by low salaries and the absence of strength of labor organizations to raise wages or improve conditions. For many African countries, this has led to a brain drain of skilled caregivers (Padarath et al., 2003). The shortage of skilled health care workers directly impacted the abilities of the provincial hospitals in this study to provide quality care. Hospitals must compete with more attractive hospitals in the public system, better paying private hospitals, and far better paying hospitals in developed countries. Again, the district hospital in the rural area that was part of this study is at the bottom of this global labor chain.

The HIV/AIDS epidemic exploded in sub-Saharan Africa against the back drop of this history. As jobs became scarce during the years of the SAPs, HIV/AIDS spread in sub-Saharan Africa along routes of labor migration and transportation (KZN DoH, 2003). Basu (2004) has pointed out how this displacement and economic struggle created a context for high-risk sexual behavior. In South Africa, stigma and denial of HIV/AIDS in the community was supported by denial of the link between HIV and AIDS, the failure to implement strong treatment and prevention policy, and a general lack of strong open leadership from the top of government. In the public hospitals, the picture was one of services overrun by people suffering from the opportunistic infections (OIs) related to HIV/AIDS (Floyd, Reid, Wilkinson, & Gilks, 1999) and specific problems caused by vast increases in morbidity and mortality. In particular, hospitals were not set up for palliative care, leading to the policy of family member/volunteer home-based care providers.

The stigma, denial, and confusion engendered by the governments' lack of official recognition of the devastation of the epidemic[1] created a strange situation,

---

[1] Governments' lack of recognition of the problem is not the sole cause of denial. But the ANC in South Africa has a very high level of authority and social influence due to its history as part of the liberation movement, so the government's role is more important than it might be in other country contexts.

in which, at the most intimate level, caregivers and patients could not talk about HIV/AIDS openly.

A labor/work-environment approach to public health is one that aligns the conditions for safe work and rights in the workplace with the importance of health care workers in providing the care, treatment, and education that is the cornerstone of health services. It begins with investments that directly impact safe working conditions and the ability of those who provide care to participate meaningfully in how care is provided.

This study found that key investments in hospitals, patients, and nurses were lacking, and that nurses were weak advocates for their own rights and the rights of patients. Background chapters showed that, far from occurring in isolation, these situations for South African nurses were consistent with worldwide trends toward privatization and commodification of health care engendered by neoliberal globalization. A labor/work-environment perspective that relies on investments in the work environment, human capacity, and public health is at odds with the neoliberal philosophy that measures success through narrow economic growth, and assumes that efficiency alone can contribute to quality in health care.

In the discussion that follows, I will discuss the results of the case study in context in light of current initiatives, policies, and social movements that hold promise for labor/work-environment improvements. A critical analysis that supports these changes rests in an analysis of the HIV/AIDS epidemic that so threatens South Africa and the nurses in this study, but which has been contributed to worldwide by people affected by the disease. This can be understood through looking at the Treatment Action Campaign(TAC) in South Africa and its role in pushing the understanding of HIV/AIDS as a social, political, and economic issue, not just a medical one.

The Industrial Health Research Group (IHRG) at the University of Cape Town (UCT) has been one of the few organizations in South Africa (and the world) that has investigated, written about, and developed interventions focused on the issue of health care workers, occupational health and HIV/AIDS, while promoting solutions that are union-based and rely on nurses collective organizing and power. In the introduction to a brochure on OHS and HIV, IHRG describes the broad issue of HIV and South African society that are the basis for shop-floor action.

> HIV/AIDS is an incurable physical illness caused by a virus that destroys the human immune system. It is a physical disease that is transmitted by physical human actions. But the virus follows lines of social weakness— it thrives on fear, denial, neglect, and ignorance. HIV and the opportunistic sicknesses associated with AIDS spread like wildfire in conditions of poverty, malnutrition, inadequate health care, violence, rape, disrespect and discrimination.
>
> The huge impact of HIV/AIDS on our population highlights lines of power and inequality in the class, cultural, racial, gender, and generation

154 / "WHO IS NURSING THEM? IT IS US."

struggles that characterize South African society. The issues that we have to consider in the fight against HIV/AIDS embrace our personal relationships, social habits, and cultural practices. We see the disease feeding on our silences, fears, and denials. We see it taking advantage of our deep economic and social inequalities. We see it thriving on our lack of political will.

We can look back in awe at the collective determination with which we fought apartheid and wonder why we stand so paralyzed today in the face of the destruction caused by HIV/AIDS. HIV/AIDS is not just a physical illness that needs medical treatment. It is a devastating social epidemic that can only be stopped through an aggressive culture of care. The development of that culture of care requires radical shifts in political, economic, social, cultural, and personal behavior. (Industrial Health Research Group [IHRG], 2003)

This quote echoes the Maputo Statement on HIV/AIDS (1990) in its scope of understanding of the causes and meaning of the epidemic. It also speaks to the question of the power of organized South Africans to make social change: why should it be that people who experienced such a recent, monumental victory should be so paralyzed by HIV/AIDS? The quote ends by prescribing the need for an "aggressive culture of care," which could be applied to health care workers and general society alike. In what follows, I will discuss the potential for this social movement in light of this case study and the global situation for health care.

Neoliberalism and the KZN Public Hospitals

I set out to look at the influence of HIV/AIDS and neoliberal globalization on the work environment of public-sector hospital nurses. At the outset, there were certain features I drew on that others have already associated with neoliberal globalization. I knew that macroeconomic policy had restricted health-sector spending in South Africa (Stack & Hlela, 2002), and that repayment of apartheid era debt reduced the level of funds available to the budget overall (Bond, 2004). Nursing shortages were a big problem in KZN, and South Africa generally, and these shortages were related to a global race to the bottom in terms of wages and working conditions for health care workers. But what did I find that strengthens the argument that neoliberalism in particular is the culprit? It would be possible to argue, for example, that the district hospital in this study was historically neglected, and simply continued to be; that there was no difference for the people who work there between 2003 and 1973, or 1923 for that matter. On the other hand, some might argue that the gleaming, paperless, central hospital run as a PPP is an inspirational victory of globalization.

However, insights gained in this study support the argument that neoliberal globalization is specifically responsible for inequities and problematic working conditions in the KZN system. At the district hospital, a cholera outbreak at the time of my visit echoed outbreaks since 2001, which were unparalleled in local history (Jeter, 2002). These were directly tied to the local authority privatization of water, which led to the practice of river water substitution. Communal taps were metered and require payment before water could be accessed. Water privatization is an example of contracting with the private sector and the principle of cost-recovery in basic services. International corporations involved in delivering water services are benefactors of neoliberalism. The cholera outbreak and its ripple effect on the hospital and patient population is a direct impact of neoliberalism and the underdevelopment of the surrounding community.

Stack and Hlela (2002) note that KZN lacked a flagship hospital, and the South African Government (RSA, 2004) notes that tertiary care services were duplicated in KZN facilities. However, the need for centralized tertiary services does not justify the disparities between the central hospital and other provincial hospitals in this study. While it is certainly the case that public sector care should include such a beautiful, high tech facility, it is problematic that behind this flagship institution lays the destitute district hospitals where many people with HIV/AIDS and TB go for care. CH is not just an experiment in the PPP model; it is a high-profile example of PPP that is touted by top-level national government figures in international forums (Manuel, 2003). It is a showpiece for the success of neoliberal models of health care. Again, there is no problem with the PPP per se, but it is telling that it offers no solutions to the dilemma of providing care to the rural poor, the most intractable problem for the KZN health system. The high-profile PPP strategy means that extraordinary efforts will be put into its success, while invisible district-level services continue to deteriorate.[2]

In an environment that is competitive for funds, expertise, DoH attention, and health workers, CH is a drain that impacts the rest of the system. Key examples are the supported recruitment activities—justified by commissioning—that pulled health workers from less attractive provincial hospitals in KZN: "Many go to the CH, they have nice flats that are subsidized. People like to go there, everything is nice there" (Ngubane, NM). The fact that there were inevitable hold-ups in commissioning meant that CH services continued to be duplicated at other hospitals (KZN Department of Health, 2003).

The district-level hospital is the point of entry for South Africa's poorest people who suffer from HIV/AIDS and TB. Investing in and focusing on high level, world-class tertiary services shows a neglect of this patient population and the people committed to providing their care.

In general, in this study of three provincial hospitals, having market value correlated with more attention and dynamism in the system. And the hospital with the greatest need, as measured by historical neglect and burden of disease and underdevelopment—the district hospital—receives the least attention in the

---

[2] These criticisms reflect a criticism of African health reforms that fail to address urban/rural equity (historic inequity) in Africa. See www.equinetafrica.org for a thorough discussion of these issues.

system. This is in direct contradiction of the goals of primary preventive care, and indicates the preeminence of neoliberal values over public health values.

It is important to not take this analysis too far. The South African public health care system is staffed by practitioners dedicated to the health of the poor, and policy initiatives and the South African constitution can support progressive change. But the overlay of private values erodes the human rights/social rights basis of a public system. It would be possible, probably necessary, for a role for the private sector in public health in South Africa. The issue becomes then, how to ensure that the public values of democratic input, comprehensive planning, and equity hold sway. The South African constitution makes access to health care a human right (RSA, 1996), and the health sector is guided by a plan that closely resembles the PHC models advocated by progressive public health advocates (RSA, 1997). Yet in implementation, if neoliberal policy ideas of privatization reign in social and economic policy, public health values will suffer.

In this study, the disparities between the three hospitals were fueled by the prioritization of economic concerns (market value and competition). Inequities in staff, physical space, department support, resources, and occupational health services were the result. This economic focus by government in policymaking was supported by the tone of public debate: the allocation of scarce resources, and the demands of the global economy that seem to preclude a range of policy options (in the words of minister of Finance Trevor Manuel, quoted earlier in this document, "The collapse of the Soviet Union, the destruction of the Berlin Wall broke the . . . revolutionary illusions of many. That very stark collapse shifted the debate very significantly" [Marais, 1999, p. 132]). The wider policy context is important, and the influence of neoliberal globalization on South African policymaking in the postapartheid era has been that the ANC-led government has acted in line with international actors such as the World Bank and the United States far more often than not (Bond, 2004a).

Neoliberalism Impacts on Denial and Stigma

Among the strongest results of the case study in this book was the finding that denial and stigma were strongly determinative of how HIV/AIDS was handled by nurses in the hospital setting. Managers and nurses both commented on the absence of open discussion between nurses and patients about HIV/AIDS, and it follows that in this context, nurses were not urging patients to be tested for HIV. This is important, because willingness to be tested for HIV/AIDS is important for prevention, and for confronting denial about the disease. This dilemma flowed from the fact that nurses themselves did not want to be tested, and this in turn related to their fear of a positive result given the lack of treatment, and the inability to demand safe sex. It also flowed from the fact that antiretroviral treatment (ART) was not available in the public sector for nurses or patients and the government's refusal to confront issues squarely and consistently. Nurses viewed

HIV/AIDS as a sexually transmitted, not occupationally acquired disease. They discussed their own risk in terms of stigma, women's disempowerment, and disgrace; not in terms of workplace rights. Policies on protecting the confidentiality of people living with HIV/AIDS (PLWA) were developed to protect the rights of individuals against discrimination. Yet in the context of stigma and denial, confidentiality policies ended up contributing to secrecy, gossip, and a fear of talking about HIV/AIDS openly.

Understanding the roots and dynamics of stigma and denial are beyond the scope and methods of this book. However, I would contend that the social impacts of neoliberal globalization also have an impact on the dilemmas of stigma and denial around HIV/AIDS in the hospital workplace. These social impacts include individualizing problems and creating burdens for women and workers who are rendered invisible.

At its base, neoliberal globalization views the behavior of people in relation to the market. It's basis is in individualism and consumerism (Friedman, 1962). For health systems, for example, one of the observed results of privatization is individualization (Turshen, 1999); meaning that as families struggle to get needs met or to compensate for absent services, problems become individualized. This individualization is explicit in the economic perspective. One argument for user fees for health services is that they decrease unnecessary utilization (moral hazard); this argument is based on economic calculations of individuals and families.

Stigma and denial of social problems are reinforced by factors that individualize problems. In this study, "coping" was used to describe individualizing problems at the individual and system level. In the privatized system, the energy of people is as individuals coping with family trauma and struggling to get needs met. Coping was frequently used by managers and nurses to describe how they were "getting by," given the strains of few resources and the demands of the HIV/AIDS epidemic: "I'm not sure how, but we're coping" (Chiliza, HM). Health systems are developed to provide care for the sick, as a matter apart from how they are financed. Coping is what those in the system do to make up for the gaps in resources and externalized social costs. The imperative to cope is strengthened by the fact that many who work in the field chose it for reasons that are linked to their social or religious beliefs, or because they have talents for care. However, coping can lead to acceptance, putting band-aids on problems rather than attacking the root cause. As a nurse in the IHRG/SAMWU/MSP project notes (IHRG 2005),

> We are often too busy to complain or to even consider OH&S issues. We take bad conditions as normal. It is a culture of sacrifice and acceptance. All of us—management, HCWs, SAMWU (the union)—are prepared to accept appalling conditions, as "normal" and therefore acceptable. The community also accepts appalling conditions. (p. 5)

Individualizing disease also turns the focus to individual behaviors. This is evident in health-belief models for HIV/AIDS prevention (Basu, 2004), which focus on education and individual behavior change. Yet nurses in this study appeared to have enough education about the transmission of the disease, the appropriate health beliefs, but lacked the power in their relationships at home and at work to protect themselves against HIV infection. This is not an issue for individual behavior change, but of collective action in the workplace, and social change that supports women's sexual rights.[3]

Neoliberal globalization specifically advocates for privatization and the reduction/elimination of public provision and funding of goods and services. Women bear additional burdens when public goods are reduced. Women provide care in the home when health care is unavailable. They spend additional time fetching water if there are no local sources. In short, when "social forms of care are withdrawn, the results are gendered" (Turshen, 1999). At the same time, this process is invisible to a system that has externalized these issues and is only concerned with what is paid for. Workers face similar struggles. Women are disproportionately engaged in the informal economy, where pay is lower and conditions worse than in formal work (Chen, Vanek, & Carr, 2004). While this work often has clear ties to the formal economy (for example, production chains that include home work), it is invisible to the system.

This case study showed a lack of recognition for the challenges that nurses face. At the system level, resources and support for meeting the needs of HIV/AIDS, including human resource aspects, was lacking. Nurses expressed the fact that they felt they were not recognized, and that their perceived employer, the government, did not care about them or about PLWA. Failure to recognize is another level of denial that reinforces the denial nurses are experiencing in the hospital.

Finally, failure to address the full social context of the epidemic—economics, gender, development, power, and inequality—supports stigma and denial. Labor migration, transportation routes, and the separation of families are shown to have created the conditions for the explosion of HIV/AIDS in southern Africa (Abdool-Karim & Abdool-Karim, 2002), yet no donor-funded interventions challenge these characteristics of the economy. Historically, donor-funded projects have usually reinforced existing power structures (Basu, 2004). For example, the Rockefeller foundation has a long tradition of funding vertical health interventions (those that focus on a single disease) that address impediments to the extraction of resources and thereby supported exploitative colonial relationships (Waitzkin, 2003).

---

[3] In the short term, it is also probably an appropriate issue for finding methods that reduce risk of sexual transmission of HIV that women can be in control of, as Stein (Susser, 2002) has argued.

Management's attitudes, which nurses associated mostly with the government (the upper echelon of their employer), were seen as adding insult to injury. Nurses pointed out that government's actions—spreading misinformation and not making treatment available (or not making heroic efforts to do so)—had led to the sense that "they just don't care," further entrenching stigma and denial: "Our government here, they tell you that AIDS is caused by poverty. So we definitely know that these people don't care (AIDS Clinic, RH)." Some nurses even saw these attitudes as explicitly cultivated by the ANC government as an excuse for not dealing with HIV/AIDS and other issues related to equality and human rights: they took the ANC failures as evidence of a group protecting its own class interests (unrecorded discussion among trade union nurse activists, 2003). Bond has written extensively about class formation in the new South Africa, noting that many ANC members form a new South African elite (Bond, 2000).

Nurses in this study indicated that they did not want to be silent, in denial, or to have AIDS and not have treatment. Some went so far as to advocate for "sanitariums" for people with HIV/AIDS, to avoid the deafening silence: "I am so tired of secrecy. We should have a hospital for HIV/AIDS, where the nurses are also HIV positive. Then no one will have to hide. We will not have this confidentiality, and we can discuss openly" (Maternity, RH). They gave every indication that recognition for their crucial jobs in fighting HIV/AIDS, treatment for themselves and patients, resources and care could help overcome denial and stigma. Far from a by-product of cultural norms of secrecy, these things were strongly tied to conditions. In fact, nurses made it clear that the secrecy and confidentiality were themselves a source of stress.

Nurses and managers interviewed for this study thought that introducing ART treatment could play a significant role in increasing reporting needlestick injuries and willingness to be tested for HIV, and thereby in reducing silence, stigma, and denial. Six months after this study took place, the national government agreed on a plan to deliver ART through the public sector. However, the positive gains of such a plan are not guaranteed; there are numerous pitfalls and dangers that threaten the potential benefits of the ART program, many of them related to the dilemmas of addressing health and equity in the context of neoliberal policy imperatives.

Antiretroviral Treatment (ART) for HIV/AIDS and Health Sector Development

McCoy et al. (2005) argue that, in order to realize long-term sustainable benefits, ART must be part of comprehensive health system development. They point to the situation in which ambitious targets for getting people onto ART are supported by large infusions of donor funds in many countries in sub-Saharan Africa, but weak and collapsing health systems are not being strengthened to support these programs. The authors draw on the history of structural adjustment and subsequent impact of neoliberalism on health policy to explain the weakness of SSA health systems. In particular, they argue that neoliberal models for health policy produce fragmentation of health services, which undermine comprehensive coordination of laboratories, testing, prevention and treatment services necessary to address a complicated epidemic and treatment modality. Finally, McCoy et al. posit that there are two choices: a vicious cycle in which ART programs weaken existing health systems and undermine their own goals, or a virtuous cycle where ART programs are the basis for a program to strengthen all health services. They conclude that this positive outcome will only occur if it is explicitly pursued, and that this pursuit will require activism from many levels of society.

These arguments place efforts to confront the HIV/AIDS epidemic in the context of ongoing health-sector development in the historical context of the SAPs and sub-Saharan Africa's position in the global economy. One important aspect of their argument is that sustainable efforts to provide ART must be based in sustainable public health systems, because HIV/AIDS is a complex disease with social, economic, and political components (Benatar, 2002; Farmer, 1999). Their analysis provides a useful outline for a labor/work-environment approach to a global public health crisis, because it is concerned with the creation of sustainable health care work environments with the capacity for input from a variety of stakeholders. What this book adds to the approach is the perspective of nurses in the work environment, which is essentially the frontlines of response to HIV/AIDS. Because occupational health and safety for health workers relates to nurses relations to patients, the conditions of work, workplace rights, and the relative power of health care workers, it is an important component of a healthy, safe, and sustainable work environment.

Treatment and Care for HIV/AIDS in the South African Public Sector

One policy with potential to reverse the negative impacts of disinvestment in the public hospitals and the pressures of the HIV/AIDS epidemic is the treatment and care plan released by the South African Government in November 2003. Providing treatment and care through an integrated national health program could improve working conditions and the quality of patient care. This plan dedicates half of its resources to strengthening the national health system in order to prepare for providing care and ARV treatment to an estimated 1.4 million by 2009. It specifies measures to recruit and retain the workforce, and calls for hiring 22,000 additional health care workers over the next 5 years (RSA, 2003a).

The value of having a universal public-sector program for HIV/AIDS treatment cannot be underestimated. It represents national control over HIV/AIDS treatment, which means much more than just delivering medicine. It means that the decisions about who to treat, medicines to use, people to employ, facilities to contract, and so on are in the public realm of decision making, subject to transparency, and linked to efforts like district-based primary health care. But the benefits of this program are not automatic. For example, the TAC has already sued the government over transparency issues (and won). In March 2005 the government announced its contractors to supply antiretroviral medicines, and revealed that they had chosen to use many brand-name suppliers for drugs, thus failing to challenge multinational drug companies (even though they are legally able to under WTO rules) or gain additional savings through generic versions of ARVs. Yet despite setbacks, the potential and access are there to fight for a say in the decisions. That is in the hard-won South African constitution. It is interesting that the other developing country that has a universal access to ARVs through the public system is Brazil—a country that also has a highly developed social movement. This indicates that there is a strong role for social movements in HIV/AIDS treatment, and by extension, public health.

This book identified potential pitfalls to the success of public-sector ART. Unless disparities between the KZN provincial hospitals are addressed, it is difficult to see how ART programs can be sustained on the scale that they are needed. The impacts of the PPP on the KZN system, the distorting effect of the "world class" central hospital on the overall system, and the skewed attention to the hospitals that are already the best off are examples of how privatization has weakened the KZN public system. These are pitfalls for the scale-up of ART in KZN.

In 2005 it was estimated that around 4,900 people were on ART in the KZN public sector, 112 of them at the regional hospital that was part of this study (RSA, 2006). While this is a hopeful step, the numbers represent only a fraction of those needing treatment. Considering the doctors, nurses, labs, administration, educators, counselors, and general supportive resources needed for a large-scale program, it is difficult to see how these things are available given the struggles to provide quality patient care that nurses and managers described.

Brain drain of health workers from SSA is identified as among the greatest challenges to health system development and to the scale-up of ART in South Africa. Since 2003 South Africa introduced a number of measures to increase public-sector nurse retention (RSA, 2006), attract nurses to rural areas where they are most needed, and mitigate the many problems with long- or short-term overseas migration. In this study nurses and managers described how nurses left for financial reasons and often returned to public-sector employment after losing seniority. Recently in KZN the DoH discussed allowing nurses to take unpaid leave to work overseas. Private companies in South Africa already employ such policies and one company, Netcare, gives nurses the option to work for up to 2 months a year in two U.K.-based projects and earn the overseas wage (Shevel, 2003). The ANC reports discussions with countries that recruit South African health workers to agree on "ground rules" for these activities. At the same time, South Africa recruits health professionals, including physicians from Cuba (a government program) and more recently nurses from India (a private-sector initiative). Intake of new nursing students has also increased. With unemployment high, it seems that there stands a good chance of new recruiting, despite working conditions.

The global labor market provides nurses from poorer, developing countries the "opportunity" to migrate to developed countries for higher wages, saving the developed country the costs of training workers, while robbing developing countries of sorely needed skilled workers and reducing the pressure on health systems in developed countries to improve wages and working conditions (Bach, 2003). Despite posturing about the poaching of African nurses, Britain (where most South African nurses migrate) has relaxed its restrictions on employment of foreign nurses in recent years (Reilly, 2003).

The General Agreement on Trade in Services (GATS) under the World Trade Organization reinforces current international migration trends. Although GATS is currently voluntary, full enactment could undercut national policies to strengthen health systems, including control over what health services are offered and how workers are trained. Under two trade rules, "market access" and "national treatment," GATS would eliminate national limits on health services and remove preferential treatment for national vs. international companies. Part of the GATS pertains to licensing restrictions; in an effort to increase their ability to "export" health workers, India has asked that the United States recognize the licensing of foreign medical personnel (Shaffer, Witzkin, Brenner, & Jasso-Aguila, 2005). In addition, researchers have pointed out that South Africa's GATS commitments actually contradict redistributive aspects of the 2004 National Health Act[4] (MSP, 2006).

As long as South African nurses and their families struggle to make ends meet, migration will persist. The notion of a race to the bottom has typically applied to factory work. Conventional wisdom holds that factories can be moved, not hospitals; we cannot put all the sick people on airplanes and fly them to the cheapest medical facility. Here, it is the health care workers who move, leaving short-staffed facilities behind. Hochschild uses the phrase "Nanny chain" to describe the international link between women who travel overseas to watch children, while their own children are cared for by other family members (Hochschild, 2000). This chain links the formal and informal economies and is mirrored in the care chain that results when nurses leave their home countries for health care work abroad (add the engineering of shortages).

Finally, the case study of nurses' occupational health found that many changes would be needed before nurses felt valued, safe, and empowered at work. As the basis for nurses' motivation to commit themselves to fighting HIV/AIDS, including supporting their willingness to be tested and encouraging patients to be tested (a prerequisite for treatment), these changes are part of what is needed for

---

[4]A little on the national health act.

a sustainable health system. These include pay, benefits, and recognition, which help recruit and retain skilled nurses; occupational health policies that address the social situation of nurses as women, caregivers, and community members; and nurses' active involvement in policymaking and implementation.

Social Movement for a Labor/Work Environment Approach to HIV/AIDS

While nurses' activism on the shop floor is the essential ingredient in making effective and appropriate health and safety policy, "breathing life into policy" as Henwood (2005) states, it must be socially supported. The burden of system change that supports a safe and decent workplace and quality care of patients cannot fall entirely on those who provide care. What elements of a social movement to strengthen the public health system and protect nurses' health on the job are in place in KZN, South Africa?

"De-Commodification," the Independent Left, and New Social Movements

In *Strategies for Social Justice Movements from Southern Africa to the United States,* Bond (2005) reviews the rich history of African anticolonial movements, and argues that Africa is far beyond much of the rest of the world, in that its own "Seattle" moment in antiglobalization protest has a 120-year history. In the specific context of postapartheid South Africa, Bond describes the emergence of an independent left (that has not yet left the ANC fold). This political context for the fight for public health links struggles for health as a human right to antiprivatization efforts and struggles from the bottom up for sustainable development. The Soweto Electricity Crisis Committee, the Environmental Justice Networking Forum, and the Landless People's Movement are examples of organizations that, along with the TAC, have challenged the ANC in struggles for social justice, human rights, and public health (Bond, 2005, p. 57).

Bond (2005) describes how these efforts, and others, are beginning to come together under a strategy of decommodification.

> The South African decommodification agenda is based on overlapping, interlocking campaigns to turn basic needs into genuine human rights including: free antiretroviral medicines to fight AIDS, at least 50 liters of free water and 1 kilowatt hour of free electricity for each individual every day, extensive land reform, prohibitions on service disconnections and evictions, free education, and a monthly basic income grant. Social movements, women's groups, churches, NGOs, and unions are all basically committed to this agenda, even if temporary divisions arise over alignments with Mbeki's ruling African National Congress. (p. 7)

Bond points out that this strategy depends in turn upon delinking from the most harmful aspects of international global capitalism, especially the control of the World Bank, IMF, and WTO over national industrial and macroeconomic policy. As nurses struggle over their conditions of work, these struggles take place in the broader community context. A social movement that prioritizes human rights in questions of supplying basic needs including health care could support nurses' struggles.

Two recent movements in KwaZulu-Natal represent how communities are organizing to reject the current status quo. Desai (2002) and Pithouse (2005) have written about community-based mass movements of poor people in KwaZulu-Natal. Poor Indians from Chatsworth and Africans from the township of Umlazi joined together to demand a reasonable flat rate for basic services from the municipality in response to growth in electric fees (Desai, 2002). In 2005 a march on the city council in Durban by over 5,000 people living in an informal settlement, to demand toilets and other basic rights, led to *Abahlali baseMjondolo*, the shack-dwellers movement (Pithouse, 2005). Both these developments point to new political formations in KwaZulu-Natal that, while they work within the existing political formations, are based on the democratic voice of those on the losing end of local government policies. They represent a truly grounded rejection of neoliberal policies, as those affected wield the "people power" (Alinsky, 1971), which is the essence of democratic change.

Global, Social Unionism for Nurses and
Other Health Care Workers

I introduced this book by discussing an international forum of health care workers looking at how current health policies were impacting workers around the world. By looking in-depth and empirically at the issues facing nurses in South Africa, this book adds to the understanding of worker/community impacts of health policy and how this is tied to international policies that govern national development. For South Africa to conquer AIDS through a strong public health system, an engagement of health care unions and shop floor representation, and activism is required. Labor migration and brain drain of health workers requires far more than an international "decade of human resources": it requires an international labor strategy that touches on the health policy and health systems development issues that affect community and the workforce. In order to stem the flow of health workers from south to north requires investing in the working conditions of health workers in every country, and this won't happen without worker/community activism.

Zwelinzima Vavi, the secretary of COSATU, was the keynote speaker at the inaugural event of the Cornell Global Labor Institute. During his speech, titled "A World to Win," Vavi connected the concepts of social unionism, international unionism, and nationally based sustainable development, and ended with a critique of the MDGs. His description both provides an analysis of the strength of South African trade unions and the challenges that face them.

> Because we know that workers are members of the society before they are workers, we have sought to integrate their struggles at the workplace with those of our communities. It is these forms of struggles that over time developed the capacity of COSATU as the all round movement that is the true voice of the marginalized. We have led struggles for decent houses, access to electricity and other basic amenities side by side with the need to pay workers a living wage and for improved working conditions. . . . It would be very difficult for any conservative government in the future to isolate COSATU because we are an integral part of the society. We believe that there is no future today for narrow trade unions that only focus on bread and butter issues instead of taking vigorously issues of members that are equally issues of the broader working class and the poor as well.
>
> COSATU is proposing that the ICFTU adopt a resolution calling for a broader discussion on development issues. We hope to start with regional processes, which would culminate in the adoption of some basic shared principles. The coming ICFTU congress is an important platform to take these debates forward. Equally important is engagement with the World Social Forum and democratic and progressive political parties and governments across the world. We need a new development path and a new world consensus on how it will be achieved. To just list global targets and hope that poor countries will achieve these in 2015 is unrealistic. (Vavi, 2004)

In this quote, Vavi identifies labor struggles with the broader struggle for national development. While this is a speech from the top, it is important in at least showing the willingness of organized labor to be part of a progressive struggle. However, the picture on the shop floor is not quite so clear.

Nurses' Involvement

In the South African context, Henwood of IHRG puts it thusly: "OH&S/HIV laws and policies cannot have meaning without HCW's breathing life into them through ownership, practice and struggle" (Henwood, 2005, p. 2). This book, like the joint project that Henwood is involved with, found that nurses (and unions) were not actively involved in OHS/HIV issues at the shop-floor level. The ward nurse at DH put it poignantly; she felt that she was failing her tasks due to inadequate staff, time, and training: "It is very difficult for me, dealing with health and safety, because I am full-time on the wards. I am not managing well. I am the chairperson for health and safety, but much of the time I spend on the wards, and this side is neglected" (Megeba, OHS). While all the resources invested at CH did not seem to be enough to substitute for the health worker "breathing life" into policies, the scarcity of time, resources, and staff in the most deprived setting implied that daily demands of coping took all available energy: conditions for implementation were absent.

This last point is quite important. One of the outstanding characteristics of South Africa compared with other African countries (and many developed countries) is the quality of their OHS legislation and policies. Many are based on ILO best practices (International Labor Organization [ILO], 2001) and include things that were only recently won through much activist effort in the United States (e.g., workers compensation for HIV/AIDS) or that are superior to privatized, individualistic systems like in the United States (e.g., the constitutional right to health care, the requirement of OHS committees in the workplace, which is part of the South African OHSA act, and the density of labor union membership). However, implementing these practices remains elusive for a number of reasons, including the entrenched social and economic inequality, lack of trade union activist OHS traditions, and a work environment where the larger political economy—as in many other places and industries—results in job security and salary taking precedence over OHS concerns.

Nurses (and some managers) suggestions about how to make the workplace safer indicate that if the economic, social, and political issues were confronted, a lot could be achieved to improve blood-exposure policy in the hospitals. While this is no easy task, thinking about the problems of occupational health this way does help to focus the problem. Particularly since South African public-sector health workers have a lot at their disposal—excellent national OHS policy, university-based technical assistance, an AIDS activist community that supports (TAC health care worker campaign), a unionized workforce, mandated workplace health and safety committees, and a rights-based constitutional guarantee of health care (for themselves and patients). The social capital and experience of "conscientizing,"[5] which are the products of South Africa's political and social past, make South Africa uniquely prepared for this kind of struggle.

Gender

One issue that should be separately examined is gender. The fact that hospital nurses are primarily female is important to the results of this study. The disproportionate risk of HIV infection faced by African women in sub-Saharan Africa has been explained largely by male/female power differentials (Susser, 2002). Nurses and managers referred to women's lack of ability to protect themselves: "Many husbands are coming from the mines with HIV, but women can't say wear a condom" (AIDS Clinic, RH); "Because of the position of African women, they are not in a position to demand safe sex. She doesn't have the authority. And I don't know of any African woman that isn't living in fear of being infected" (West, HM). In South Africa and elsewhere, the work that nurses do has traditionally been classified as "women's work," and nurses have

---

[5]"Conscientization" is a word that is widely used in South Africa for the process of developing political awareness through experience.

suffered the dual discrimination of wage differentials and the undervaluing of caring labor in the formal economy. Within the hierarchy of the hospital, nurses have had low status relative to doctors and managers (Marks, 1994). At the same time, HIV/AIDS has led to informalization of health care work due to policies such as home-based care. Family members and volunteers are relied upon to provide care; this supports nurses' short-staffed work in the hospital, and saps the ability of these people to participate in productive activities.

The gender dynamics of occupational risk of HIV described by nurses in this study suggest that nurses see themselves as women first and at-risk workers second. This is reflected by nurses' comments that they will be blamed for the exposure and will have their fidelity and sexual behavior questioned despite occupational risk: "Once you have the disease, it won't be seen as that you got the disease from the patient, it won't be seen that I've got it from my husband, the whole family, everyone, will think I was cheating" (Medicine, CH).

Nurses were comparatively weak in their ability to impact their working conditions; they aren't a part of developing and implementing OHS policies in the workplace. This has a historical basis. Nurses are trained to work in a highly regimented environment with almost militaristic subservience (Marks, 1994). While this has been challenged somewhat by nurses role in trade unions, trade unions in health care have had a role limited to political rights and health advocacy in the apartheid era, and bread-and-butter issues in the current era. While there were periodic fights for improved working conditions, these have not occurred in any wide-scale manner that is related to patient care. Public-sector unions are not led by nurses. DENOSA, the former nurses association, has been in an intense process of internal transformation, from a racist nonrepresentational organization, and some have complained that this has led to slowness to deal with shop-floor issues (Dlamini, SW). Others have complained that DENOSA has the same characteristic splits that have been seen in other nurses unions that combine collective bargaining and professional association. A nurse manager in this study called DENOSA a "sissy" union: "Are nurses active in the union? No, they are just paying dues. I don't know if the problem is with DENOSA or with the nurses. They don't participate. There is nothing I can see that DENOSA is contributing to the nurse's welfare. They choose it because they have to have a union,[6] not because they are getting any help. DENOSA is a sissy organization, it doesn't have any teeth (Ngubane, NM)."

Perhaps this view of the nurses unions may have changed in response to the 2007 public-sector workers strike. On June 1, 2007, nurses joined other public-sector workers in a historic 28-day strike, which shut down hospitals and other

---

[6]Since the late 1990s, nurses have been required to contribute to collective bargaining. Negsi refers to the fact that nurses have to belong to one, because nurses must pay whether they are part of a union or not.

vital services. In September, nurses won long overdue wage increases (Independent On-Line [IOL], 2007).

Collective Action for a Culture of Care:
Organizing around occupational health and HIV/AIDS

The relationship between occupational health for nurses and the neglect and social stigma of HIV/AIDS found here supports the findings of the joint project between the Industrial Health Research Group (IHRG) at the University of Cape Town, the South African Municipal Workers Union (SAMWU) and the Municipal Services Project (MSP), "Who Cares for Caregivers?" This project took place in municipal clinics and engaged a range of health workers. After looking at health and safety committees, election of health and safety representatives, workplace OHS activities, and factors concerning the capacity of municipal clinics to deal with HIV/AIDS and protect workers, participants concluded that compliance with OHS regulations and policies were minimal, there was little in the way of prevention activities, and nurses were uninvolved and poorly represented.

Yet the project identified strengths and potential through its participatory methods. As a union-based project, WCFC recognizes that change at work relies on the collective action of nurses. Thus, nurses' comparative weakness, a key finding of this book is directly addressed by the challenge to create an aggressive culture of care that requires *radical shifts in political, economic, social, cultural, and personal behavior.*

Most important for this discussion, this project used occupational health as the lens to focus nurses' issues and saw nurses caring for themselves and their patients as key to accessing their strengths in the fight for health in a vastly unequal South Africa. In very concrete ways, occupational health training of nurse representatives, which includes a strong focus on workplace rights and public health, is a tangible step toward building this strength among nurses.

> While our findings on the state of OH&S in the municipal health sector reveal a culture of neglect, the activity of the research programme initiated an alternative to that neglect. As activist investigators, the participant researchers in this programme not only explored the prevailing attitudes, behaviours, and practices of OH&S, but in doing so, began to challenge the silence and neglect that characterises that culture.
>
> Our research activity (asking questions; identifying workplace hazards; documenting case studies of workplace injury and illness; interviewing management and workers in the clinics; sharing stories of needle-prick incidents; interrogating policy and protocols; challenging employers' non-compliance; discovering rights and responsibilities; and examining the representivity and functioning of health and safety committees) constituted an organised effort to build an alternative vocal, assertive, and dynamic culture of OH&S.

However small and tentative, an important outcome of this programme has been the transformative impact that participatory action research has had, and can have on the culture of OH&S in the municipal health clinics. The possibilities opened up by this programme, present exciting challenges to SAWMU in its organisation of health workers in municipal clinics. (IHRG/SAMWU/MSP, 2005, pp. 5-6)

CHAPTER CONCLUSION: RECOMMENDATIONS FOR A LABOR/WORK ENVIRONMENT APPROACH TO PUBLIC HEALTH

A labor/work environment approach to public health relies on investments in a safe work environment and the meaningful participation of health care workers. In a larger sense, it relies on what Wooding and Levenstein call a movement for "social health." Based on the case study in this book, conditions for safe work and nurses' participation are both lacking. Based on the background section, where I described how neoliberalism has come to dominate efforts at national development, a movement for social health faces formidable obstacles. Management's control over hazards and the work environment is undermined by the influences of global capitalism on health policy, indicating that workers' struggles need to adjust their targets.

Despite the stated commitment to delivering treatment for HIV/AIDS, international efforts are rife with contradictions. Perhaps most glaring is the continued commitment to privatization, which, through the SAPs and subsequent programs in Africa, has caused disinvestment and deterioration of access to health services. Though the policy names have changed over the years, and organizations have attempted to distance themselves from the SAPs, policy initiatives have remained essentially the same—in line with the objectives of neoliberal globalization. These same priorities are reflected in the MDGs for health. Focus on workers and employment is a glaring omission of these efforts. The new focus on human resources for health takes the workforce into consideration, but doesn't deal adequately with the political and economic constraints on power.

A labor/work-environment approach to a public health crisis is one that recognizes that the health, safety, and well-being of workers are central to confronting health crises, HIV/AIDS in particular. Care, treatment, prevention, and education must be provided by a motivated and supported workforce, something that increased donor funds and high-level conferences can't replace. While all efforts to protect workers are positive, there is no substitute for the workforces own involvement in making and implementing policy. Policies will not be implemented effectively if nurses don't breathe life into them; and this breath, in turn, is vital to the life of health systems.

APPENDIX

ℭ℘ ℘ℭ

Group Interview Results Summary

In Boxes 1, 2, and 3, highlighted items represent opinions that are nearly unanimous (at least eight of nine nurses agree) among nurses in group interviews. The other items in these lists were mentioned by more than one nurse and agreed upon by nodding and discussion in a majority (at least six of nine) of the nine groups interviewed.

**Box 1: Workplace Exposure:
Feedback from Group Interviews with Hospital Nurses**

How and why does accidental exposure to HIV most typically occur?

- Disposal of needle
- Injection
- Suturing (maternity only)
- Child birth (maternity only)
- Violent/agitated patients
- Carelessness
- Short-staffing
- Lack of appropriate training for procedure

Why do needlesticks and accidental exposures go unreported by nurses?

- Don't want to know HIV status
- Lack of confidentiality of test result
- HIV testing alone results in stigma
- Humiliating reporting process
- Do not want to take PEP
- Nurses blamed for the exposure
- No treatment available

What are the attitudes and beliefs of nurses toward PEP?

- ARV drugs make you sick
- Most nurses do not complete PEP treatment
- Required blood testing to determine status of nurse is a deterrent to PEP
- General knowledge of the need for timely initiation of PEP

How do nurses evaluate protective equipment?

- Gloves most identified for protection
- Amount and nature of protection offered by gloves not known
- Gloves not always worn
- Poor quality gloves
- Goggles and aprons unavailable
- Confusion over needle disposal policy
- Protective gear makes patients feel stigmatized
- Treating each patient as if HIV+ is unrealistic given lack of protective equipment and other resources

Box 2: Impacts of HIV on Nursing:
Feedback from Group Interviews with Hospital Nurses

How has HIV/AIDS epidemic changed who nurses care for?

• Increase in the number of HIV/AIDS patients
• Increase in the number of TB patients
• Sicker patients
• Younger patients
• "Non-clinic" mothers (no prenatal care)

How has HIV/AIDS changed relations between nurse and patient?

• Nurse maintains confidentiality between family members
• Difficulty administering neviripine at birth while maintaining confidentiality of patient status
• Hard to answer questions about PMTCT and ARV treatment
• Protective measures distance nurse from patient, seem stigmatizing

What sources of stress do nurses attribute to the HIV/AIDS epidemic?

• Fear of infection
• Overwork
• HIV+ coworkers stigmatized
• Depressing environment
• Poor working conditions
• Family pressure to quit job
• Lack of recognition of workplace exposure as source of HIV infection
• Community prevalence
• Contradictions between community ideas and workplace ideas about HIV/AIDS

What is the impact of HIV/AIDS on hospital staffing?

• Short-staffed due to poor working conditions
• Nurses leave for jobs abroad
• Retired nurses hired on contract basis to fill gaps

**Box 3: Workplace and Government Policies:
Feedback from Group Interviews with Hospital Nurses**

How do nurses evaluate hospital and DoH policy?

- Patients' rights are respected, but not nurses'
- Policy is written for hospital not nurse's benefit
- Forms are too extensive and confusing
- Protective equipment is not available

Why do nurses feel undervalued by their employer?

- Underpaid
- Pay and benefits not commensurate with other high-risk public-sector jobs
- Under recognized
- Blamed rather than supported

How do nurses view government's response to HIV/AIDS?

- Lack of treatment a huge problem
- Government lacks commitment, promotes denial
- Comments from government that poverty/poor nutrition cause AIDS are harmful

---

CR SO

References

Abdool-Karim, Q., & Abdool-Karim, S. S. (2002). The evolving HIV epidemic in South Africa. *International Journal of Epidemiology, 31*(1), 37-40.

Abdool-Karim, S. (2002, May). Interview, University of Natal Durban.

Adelzadeh, A. (1996). *From the RDP to GEAR: The gradual embracing of neoliberalism in economic policy*. National Institute of Economic Policy, South Africa.

Aiken L. H., Sloane D. M., & Klocinski, J. L. (1997). Hospital nurses' occupational exposure to blood: Prospective, retrospective and institutional reports. *American Journal of Public Health, 87*(1),103-107.

African National Congress (ANC). (1955). Freedom charter. Adopted at the Congress of the People, Kliptown, on 26 June 1955. [retrieved on February 21, 2004] Available from: http://www.anc.org.za/ancdocs/history/charter.html

African National Congress (ANC). (1992). *Reconstruction and development programme.* Johannesburg: Umanyano Publications.

African National Congress (ANC). (2002). Address at the Opening of Inkosi Albert Luthuli Central Hospital, November 22 by Vice President Jacob Zuma. [retrieved on February 21, 2005] Available from: http://www.anc.org.za/ancdocs/history/zuma/2002/jz1122.html

Akintola, O. (2004). *The gendered burden of home-based care-giving.* Durban: Health Economic and HIV/AIDS Research Division. Available from: www.heard.org.za

Alinsky, S. (1971). *Rules for radicals: A pragmatic printer for realistic radicals.* New York: Vintage Books.

Arhin-Tenkorang, D. (2000). *Mobilizing resources for health: The case for user fees revisited. Commission on Macroeconomic and Health Working Paper Series,* paper no. WG3:6. World Health Organization. [retrieved on September 14, 2004] Available from: www.cmhealth.org/docs/wg3_paper6.pdf

Arrighi G. (2002). The African crisis: World systemic and regional aspects. *New Left Review, 15,* 5-36.

Azaroff, L. S., Levenstein, C., & Wegman, D. (2002). Occupational injury and illness surveillance: Conceptual filters explain underreporting. *American Journal of Public Health, 92,* 1421-1429.

Bach, S. (2003). *International migration of health workers: Labour and social issues.* Sectoral activities working paper: WP.209. Geneva: International Labor Organization.

[retrieved on January 12, 2005] Available from: www.ilo.org/public/english/dialogue/sector/papers/health/wp209.pdf

Banerji, D. (1984). Primary health care: Selective or comprehensive? *World Health Forum, 5,* 312-315.

Banerji, D. (1999). A fundamental shift in the approach to international health by WHO, UNICEF, and the World Bank: Instances of the practice of "intellectual fascism" and totalitarianism in some Asian countries. *International Journal of Health Services, 29*(2), 227-259.

Banerji, D. (2004). The people and health service development in India: A brief overview. *International Journal of Health Services, 34*(1), 123-142.

Barnett, T., & Whiteside, A. (2002). *AIDS in the twenty-first century.* New York: Palgrave Macmillan.

Basu, S. (2004). AIDS, empire, and public health behaviorism. *International Journal of Health Services, 34*(1), 155-167.

Bateman, C. (2001). Can KwaZulu-Natal hospitals cope with the HIV AIDS human tide? *South African Medical Journal, 91*(5), 364-368.

Bates, R. (1981). *Markets and agriculture: The political basis of agriculture policy.* Berkeley: University of California Press.

Benatar, S. R. (2001). South Africa's transition in a globalizing world: HIV/AIDS as a window and a mirror. *International Affairs, 77*(2), 347-375.

Benatar, S. R. (2002). The HIV/AIDS pandemic: A sign of instability in a complex global system. *The Journal of Medicine and Philosophy, 27*(2), 163-177.

Benatar, S. R. (2004). Health care reform and the crisis of HIV and AIDS in South Africa. *New England Journal of Medicine, 351*(1), 81-92.

Berg, E. (1981). *Accelerated development in sub-Saharan Africa.* Washington DC: World Bank.

Berkman, A., Garcia, J., Munoz-Laboy, M., Paiva, V., & Parker, R. (2005). A critical analysis of the Brazilian response to HIV/AIDS: Lessons learned for controlling and mitigating the epidemic in developing countries. *American Journal of Public Health, 95*(7), 1162-1174.

Bond, P. (1999). Globalization, pharmaceutical pricing, and South African health policy: Managing confrontation with U.S. firms and politicians. *International Journal of Health Services, 29*(4), 765-792.

Bond, P. (2000). *Elite transition: From apartheid to neo-liberalism in South Africa.* London: Pluto Press.

Bond, P. (2003). *Against global apartheid: South Africa meets the World Bank, IMF and international finance.* Cape Town: University of Cape Town Press.

Bond, P. (2004a). The political roots of South Africa's cholera epidemic. In M. Fort, M. A. Mercer, & O. Gish (Eds.), *Sickness and wealth: The corporate assault on global health* (pp. 119-130). Cambridge, MA: South End Press.

Bond, P. (2004b). South Africa's frustrating decade of freedom: From racial to class V apartheid. *Monthly Review, 55*(10), 45-59.

Bond, P. (2005). Strategies for social justice movements from South Africa to the United States. Foreign Policy in Focus. Silver City, NM & Washington, DC: Foreign Policy in Focus, January 20. Available from: http://www.fpif.org/papers/0501movements_body.html

Bond, P., Dor, G., & Ruiters, G. (2000). Transformation in Infrastructure Policy from Apartheid to Democracy. Municipal Services Project, background series. Graduate School of Public and Development Management, University of Witwatersrand, Johannesburg. Available from: http://www.queensu.ca/msp/

Brannon, R. L. (1994). *Intensifying care: The hospital industry, professionalization, and the reorganization of the nursing labor process.* New York: Baywood.

Brown, G. (2004, April 8). *Vulnerable workers in the global economy. Occupational hazards.* [retrieved on September 7, 2004] Available from: http://www.occupational hazards.com/articles/11630

Brown, G. (2007, June 15). *Taking a closer look. Occupational hazards.* [retrieved on July 10, 2009] Available from: www.occupationalhazards.com/issue/Article/66378/ Taking_a_closer_lookaspx

Burawoy, M., Blum, J. A., George, S., Zsuzsa, G., Thayer, M., Gowan, T., et al. (2000). *Global ethnography: Forces, connections, and imaginations in a post-modern world.* Berkeley: University of California Press.

Centers for Disease Control (CDC). (1987). Recommendations for prevention of HIV transmission in health-care settings. *MMWR Recommendations and Reports, 36*(Suppl 2S), 3-18.

Centers for Disease Control (CDC). (2001). Updated U.S. Public Health Service guidelines for the management of occupational exposures to HBV, HCV, and HIV and recommendations for postexposure prophylaxis. *MMWR, Recommendations and Reports, 50*(RRl1), 1-42.

Chang, G. (2000). *Disposable domestics: Immigrant workers in the global economy.* Cambridge, MA: South End Press.

Chen, L., Evans, T., Anand, S., Bouffard, J. I., Brown, H., Chowdhury, M., et al. (2004). Human resources for health: Overcoming the crisis. *Lancet, 364,* 1984-1990.

Chen, M. A., Vanek, J., & Carr, M. (2004). Mainstreaming informal employment and gender in poverty reduction: A handbook for policy-makers and other stakeholders. United Kingdom: Commonwealth Secretariat/IDRC.

Chihaa, Y. A., & Link, C. R. (2003). The shortage of registered nurses and some new estimates of the effects of wages on registered nurses labor supply: A look at the past and a preview of the 21st century. *Health Policy, 64*(3), 349-375.

Clarke, S. P., Sloane, D. M., & Aiken, L. H. (2002). Effects of hospital staffing and organizational climate on needlestick injuries to nurses. *American Journal of Public Health, 92*(7), 1115-1119.

Colvin, M., Dawood, S., Kleinschmidt, I., Mullick, S., & Lallo, U. (2001). Prevalence of HIV and HIV-related diseases in the adult medical wards of a tertiary hospital in Durban, South Africa. *International Journal of STD & AIDS, 12*(6), 386-389.

Colvin, M., Gumede, L., Grimwade, K., Maher, D., & Wilkinson, D. (2003). Contribution of traditional healers to a rural tuberculosis control programme in Hlabisa, South Africa. *International Journal of Tuberculosis and Lung Disease, 7*(9 Suppl), S86-S91.

Congress of South African Trade Unions. (2000). Accelerating transformation. *The Shopsteward, 9*(3). [retrieved on August 17, 2004] Available from: http://www.cosatu. org.za/shop/shop0903/shop0903-02.htm

Connelly, P. (2005). Boston University School of Public Health. Personal correspondence.

Coovadia, H. M. (2002, April). Nelson Mandela School of Medicine; Centre for HIV/AIDS Networking (HIVAN). Interview.

Corbett, E., Steketee, R., O Ter Kuile, F., Latif, A. S., Kamali, A., & Hayes, R. (2002). HIV/AIDS and the control of other infectious diseases in Africa. *Lancet, 359,* 2177-2187.

Crush, J., Peberdy, S., Williams, V., & Southern African Migration Project (SAMP). (2006). *International migration and good governance in the Southern African Region Migration Policy Brief No. 17.* [retrieved on July 12, 2009] Available from: http://www.queensu.ca/samp/sampresources/samppublications/policybriefs/brief17.pdf

Cullinan, K. (2004, May 17). KwaZulu-Natal struggling to keep up. Health e news service. [retrieved on February 14, 2005] Available from: http://www.health-e.org.za/news/article.php?uid=20030999

D'Adesky, A. C. (2004). *Moving mountains: The race to treat global AIDS.* London: Verso.

Daily News (SA). (2000, April 13). [editorial] *Violence still upsetting health care in KZN. A hospital in KZN battles to continue in the face of crime and violence.* [retrieved on January 17, 2004] Available from: www.hst.co.za/news/item.php?nws_id=20000414

Davis, P., & Fort, M. (2004). The battle against global AIDS. In M. Fort, M. A. Mercer, & O. Gish (Eds.), *Sickness and wealth: The corporate assault on global health* (pp. 145-157). Cambridge, MA: South End Press.

Desai, A. (2002). *We are the poors: Community struggles in post-apartheid South Africa.* New York: Monthly Review Press.

Durban Declaration, The. (2000). *Nature, 406,* 15-16. [retrieved on June 26, 2008] Available from: http://www.nature.com/nature/journal/v406/n6791/full/406015a0.html

Epstein, S. (1996). *Empire science: AIDS, activism, and the politics of science.* Berkeley: University of California Press.

Farmer, P. (1999). *Infections and inequalities: The modern plagues.* Berkeley: University of California Press.

Farmer, P., Léandre, F., Mukherjee, J. S., Claude, M., Nevil, P., Smith-Fawzi, M. C., et al. (2001). Community-based approaches to HIV treatment in resource-poor settings. *Lancet, 358*(9279), 404-409.

Floyd, K., Reid, R. A., Wilkinson, D., & Gilks, C. F. (1999). Admission trends in a rural South African hospital during the early years of the HIV epidemic. *Journal of the American Medical Association, 282*(11), 1087-1091.

Folbre, N., Bergmann, B., Floro, M., & Agarwal, B. (Eds.). (1991). *Issues in contemporary economics Vol. 4: Women's work in the world economy.* London: Macmillan.

Fonn, S., & Xaba, M. (2001). Health workers for change: Developing the initiative. *Health Policy and Planning, 16*(suppl. 1), 13-18.

Fort, M. (2004). Globalization and health. In M. Fort, M. A. Mercer, & O. Gish (Eds.), *Sickness and wealth: The corporate assault on global health* (pp. 1-8). Cambridge, MA: South End Press.

Fourie, B., & Weyer, K. (2002). *Tuberculosis Research Lead Programme, MRC, Durban, South Africa.* Unpublished data.

Friedman, M. (1962). *Capitalism and freedom.* Chicago, IL: University of Chicago Press.

Friedman, S., & Mottiar, S. (2004). *Rewarding engagement?: The Treatment Action Campaign and the politics of HIV/AIDS. Globalization, marginalization and new social movements in post-apartheid South Africa.* Centre for Civil Society, School of Development Studies. University of KwaZulu-Natal, Durban. Available from: http://www.ukzn.ac.za/ccs/

Geiger, H. J. (2002). Community-oriented primary care: A path to community development. [Historical Article. Journal Article] *American Journal of Public Health, 92*(11), 1713-1716.

Gerberding, J. L. (1995). Prophylaxis for occupational exposure to bloodborne viruses. *New England Journal of Medicine, 332,* 444-455.

Gerberding, J. (2003). Occupational exposure to HIV in health care settings. *New England Journal of Medicine, 348,* 826-833.

Gish, O. (2004). The legacy of colonial medicine. In M. Fort, M. A. Mercer, & O. Gish (Eds.), *Sickness and wealth: The corporate assault on global health* (pp. 19-26). Cambridge, MA: South End Press.

Gloyd, S. (2004). Sapping the poor: The impact of structural adjustment programs. In M. Fort, M. A. Mercer, & O. Gish (Eds.), *Sickness and wealth: The corporate assault on global health* (pp. 43-54). Cambridge, MA: South End Press.

Gounden, Y. P., & Moodley, J. (2000). Exposure to human immunodeficiency virus among healthcare workers in South Africa. *International Journal of Gynaecology and Obstetrics, 69*(3), 265-270.

Gumodoka, B., Favot, I., Berege, Z. A., & Dolmans, W. M. (1997). Occupational exposure to the risk of HIV infection among health care workers in Mwanza Region, United Republic of Tanzania. *Bulletin of World Health Organization, 75*(2), 133-140.

Habib, A., & Padayachee, V. (2000). Economic policy and power relations in South Africa: Economic, social and health transformation in question. *World Development, 28*(2), 1-33.

Hanrahan, A., & Reutter, L. (1997). A critical review of the literature on sharps injuries: Epidemiology, management of exposures and prevention. *Journal of Advanced Nursing, 25*(1), 144-154.

Harrison, A., Wilkinson, D., Lurie, M., Connoly, A. M., & Abdool-Karim, S. S. (1998). Improving quality of sexually transmitted disease case management in rural South Africa. *AIDS, 12,* 2329-2335.

Health Systems Trust (HST). (2004). *Health statistics, population by province.* [retrieved on December 3, 2004]. Available from: http://www.hst.org.za/healthstats/3/data

Henwood, N., & Industrial Health Research Group. (2005). South Africa's Industrial Health Research Group comments. *Journal of Public Health Policy, 26*(2), 186-191.

Heywood, M. (2005). The price of denial. *Treatment Action Campaign* electronic newsletter, Mar 14. [retrieved on March 31, 2005] Available from: http://www.tac.org.za/home.htm

Hochschild, A. (2000). The nanny chain. *The American Prospect, 11*(4): 87-99.

Hong, E. (2004). The primary health care movement meets the free market. In M. Fort, M. A. Mercer, & O. Gish (Eds.), *Sickness and wealth: The corporate assault on global health* (pp. 27-42). Cambridge, MA: South End Press.

Horsman, J. M., & Sheeran, P. (1995). Health care workers and HIV/AIDS: A critical review of the literature. *Social Science and Medicine, 41*(11),1535-1567.

Huddart, J., & Picazo, O. A. (2003). The health sector human resource crisis in Africa: An issues paper. United States Agency for International Development, Bureau for Africa, Office of Sustainable Development Washington, DC.

IDASA, Institute for Democracy in Africa, AIDS Budget Unit. (2004). Funding the fight: Budgeting for HIV/AIDS in developing countries. [retrieved on June 19, 2009] Available from: http://www.google.com/cse?q=south+africa+HIV%2FAIDS+2003+budget&cx=011398949797700025820%3Aoaunv7w6b-e&ie=UTF-8

Independent On-Line [IOL]. (2007, September 14). Nurses will be paid more. Published on the world wide web by the Independent Online (IOL), 18:22:50. Available from: http://www.iol.co.za/general/news/newsprint.php?art_id=nw200709. Accessed on November 16, 2007.

Industrial Health Research Group. (2003). HIV/AIDS booklet, draft. Unpublished. IHRG, University of Cape Town.

Industrial Health Research Group. (2005). *Who cares for health care workers?* Final report on the SAMWU/MSP/IHRG Municipal Health Sector Occupational Health and Safety and HIV/AIDS Training and Research Programme of 2003/4. Cape Town: IHRG.

International Labor Organization. (2001). *An ILO code of practice on HIV/AIDS and the world of work.* Geneva: International Labor Office.

Irwin, A., Millen, J., & Fallows, D. (2003). *Global AIDS: Myths and facts.* Cambridge, MA: South End Press.

Jeter, J. (2002, November/December). *South Africa's driest season: The government's push to lure private companies to buy its utilities has led to water shutoffs and the worst cholera epidemic in the nation's history—The price of water.* Mother Jones. Foundation for National Progress.

Joint Learning Initiative (JLI). (2004). *Human resources for health: Overcoming the crisis.* Cambridge, MA: Global Equity Initiative, Harvard University.

Johnstone, P. (1994). *Success while others fail: Social movement unionism and the public workplace.* Ithaca, NY: ILR Press.

Kark, S. L., & Cassel, J. (2002). The Pholela Health Centre: A progress report. 1952. [Biography. Classical Article. Historical Article. Journal Article] *American Journal of Public Health, 92*(11), 1743-1747.

Kark, S. L., & Kark, E. (1983). An alternative strategy in community health care: Community-oriented primary health care. [Journal Article] *Israel Journal of Medical Sciences, 19*(8), 707-713.

Kim, J. Y., Millen, J., Irwin, I., & Gershman, J. (Eds.). (2000). Dying for growth: Global inequality and the health of the poor. Monroe, ME: Common Courage Press.

KwaZulu Natal Provincial Government. (2001). Policy and procedural protocol to be followed following accidental exposure to HIV and Hepatitis B. KZN Department of Health. [retrieved December 3, 2004] Available from: http://www.kznhealth.gov.za/occhealth/cirG70.2001.pdf

KwaZulu Natal Provincial Government. (2002). KZN Department of Health Annual Report 2001-2002. [retrieved on March 16, 2004] Available from: http://www.kznhealth.gov.za/

KwaZulu Natal Provincial Government. (2003). KZN Department of Health Annual Report 2002/2003. Available from: http://www.kznhealth.gov.za/annualreport2002.2003.pdf

KwaZulu Natal Provincial Government. (2003). KZN Provincial Treasury Department Budget statement 1, 2003. Available from: www.treasury.gov.za/.../Budget%20Statements/MPU/MPU%20-%20Budget%20Statement%201%20-%20Budget%20Overview.pdf

Loewenson, R. (1993). Structural adjustment and health policy in Africa. *International Journal of Health Services, 23*(4), 717-731.

Loewenson R. (1999). Women's occupational health in globalization and development. *American Journal of Industrial Medicine, 36,* 34-42.

Loewenson, R. (2001). Globalization and occupational health: A perspective from Southern Africa. *Bulletin of the World Health Organization, 79*(9), 863-868.

MacGillis, D. (2004). An AIDS brain drain. *The Boston Globe,* Jul 23; Sect. A:20.

Manuel, T. (2003, April 16). *Development and human rights: The South African experience,* Ames Courtroom, Harvard Law School. Co-Sponsored by the W.E.B. Du Bois Institute, the Committee on African Studies, and the Human Rights Program.

Marais, H. (1999). *South Africa limits to change: The political economy of transition.* London: Zed Books, Ltd.

Marks, S. (1994). *Divided sisterhood: Race, class and gender in the South African nursing profession.* New York: St. Martins Press.

Marks, S. (2002). An epidemic waiting to happen? The spread of HIV/AIDS in sociological and historical perspective. *African Studies, 61*(1), 13-27.

Martinez, J., & Martineau, T. (1998). Rethinking human resources: An agenda for the millennium. *Health Policy and Planning, 13*(4), 345-358.

Mashaba, T. G. (1995). *Rising to the challenge: A history of black nursing in South Africa.* Cape Town: Juta & Co.

Mast, S. T., Woolwine, J. D., & Gerberding, J. L. (1993). Efficacy of gloves in reducing blood volumes transferred during simulated needlestick injury. *Journal of Infectious Diseases, 168,* 1589-1592.

McCoy, D., Chopra, M., Loewenson, R., Aitken, J. M., Ngulube, T., Muula, A. et al. (2005). Expanding access to antiretroviral therapy in sub-Saharan Africa: Avoiding pitfalls and dangers, capitalizing on opportunities. *American Journal of Public Health, 95*(1), 18-22.

McDonald, O., & Ruiters, G. (Eds.). (2005, January). *Who cares for health workers? The state of occupational health and safety in municipal clinics in South Africa.* Industrial Health Research Group and the South African Municipal Workers Union. Municipal Services Project, Occasional paper series No. 8.

McMichael, P. (2000). *Development and social change: A global perspective* (2nd ed.). Thousand Oaks, CA: Pine Forge Press.

McNeill, P. (2002, May). Port Shepstone Hospital, KwaZulu-Natal South Africa. Interview.

Melosch, B. (1982). *"The physician's hand": Work culture and conflict in American nursing.* Philadelphia, PA: Temple University Press.

Millen, J., & Holtz, T. (2000). Dying for growth Part 1: Transnational corporations and the health of the poor. In J. Y. Kim, J. Millen, I. Irwin, & J. Gershman (Eds.), *Dying for growth: Global inequality and the health of the poor* (pp. 177-224). Monroe, ME: Common Courage Press.

Mkandawire, T., & Soludo, C. (1999). *Our continent our future: African perspectives on structural adjustment.* Trenton, NJ: African World Press, Inc.

Moody, K. (1998). *An injury to all: The decline of American unionism.* New York: Verso.

Moore, S. (2003). Unrelenting tide of AIDS erodes burial traditions. *Los Angeles Times,* Jan. 12; Sect. A:6. Available from: http://www.hst.org.za/news/20030124

Municipal Services Project (MSP). (2009). Project objectives. [retrieved on November 13, 2009] Available at www.municipalservicesproject.org/about-us/project-objectives

Muntaner, C., & Lynch, J. (2002). Income inequality, social cohesion, and class relations: A critique of Wilkinson's neo-Durkheimian research program. In V. Navarro (Ed.), *The political economy of social inequalities: Consequences for health and quality of life.* Amityville, NY: Baywood.

Myers, J. E., & Macun, I. (1989). The sociologic context of occupational health in South Africa. *American Journal of Public Health, 79*(2), 216-224.

Myers, J. E., & Macun, I. (1993). New developments in South African health and safety legislation. *South African Medical Journal, 83*(1), 1.

Nathan, E. (2004). Partnerships boost Africa's development. *Business Day,* August 11, 2004. [retrieved on March 2, 2005] Available from: http://www.bday.co.za/bday/content/direct/1,3523,1677014-6078-0,00.html

Navarro, V. (2004). The world situation and the WHO. *Lancet, 363,* 1321-1324.

Ncayiyana, D. J. (2004). Doctors and nurses with HIV and AIDS in sub-Saharan Africa. *British Medical Journal, 329*(7466), 584-585.

Ntuli, A. (Ed.). (2001). South African Health Review 2001. Durban: Health Systems Trust. Available from: http://www.hst.org.za/publications/481

Nyerere, J. K. (1979, February 12). *Unity for a new order.* Address by President Julius K. Nyerere to the Ministerial Conference of the Group of 77, Arusha, Tanzania. [retrieved August 12, 2004] Available from http://www.southcentre.org/mwalimu/speeches/written/unityforaneworder/mwalimuspeech.htm

O'Donnell, M., & Zelnick, J. (2002). *The AIDS/tuberculosis epidemic in KwaZulu-Natal: Opportunities for action.* Policy Brief commissioned by HIV/AIDS Education and Research Division (HEARD), University of Natal, Durban for the KwaZulu-Natal Department of Health.

Ofili, A. N., Asuzu, M. C., & Okojie, O. H. (2003). Hospital workers' opinions on the predisposing factors to blood-related work accidents in Central Hospital, Benin City, Edo State, Nigeria. *Public Health, 117*(5), 333-338.

Organization of African Unity (OAU). (1980). Lagos plan of action for the economic development of Africa, 1980-2000. [retrieved on August 15, 2004] Available from: http://www.uneca.org/itca/ariportal/docs/lagos_plan.pdf

Orr, L., Heintz, J., & Tregenna, F. (1998). *A gendered critique of GEAR.* National Labor and Economic Development Institute. Johannesburg: NALEDI.

Padarath, A., Chamberlain, C., McCoy, D., Ntuli, A., Rowson, M., & Loewenson, R. (2003). Health personnel in Southern Africa: Confronting maldistribution and brain drain. Equinet Discussion Paper Number 4, Equinet Policy Series. [retrieved on June 5, 2004] Available from: http://www.equinetafrica.org/Resources/downloads/HRH%20Review.pdf

Parker, R. (2003). Building the foundations for the response to HIV/AIDS in Brazil: The development of HIV/AIDS policy, 1982-1996. *Divulgacao em Saude para Debate, Rio de Janeiro 27,* 143-183.

People's Budget Campaign. (2004). *People's budget response to the 2003 medium term budget policy statement.* COSATU/SANGOCO/SACC. [retrieved on December 15, 2004] Available from: www.naledi.org.za

People's Budget Campaign. (2005-2006). *People's budget.* A proposal from COSATU, SANGOCO, and SACC. National Labor and Economic Development Institute. Johannesburg; NALEDI; 2004. [retrieved on March 15, 2005] Available from: http://www.naledi.org.za/docs/Peoples-Budget-Title.pdf

Phaladze, N. A. (2003). The role of nurses in the human immunodeficiency virus/acquired immune deficiency syndrome policy process in Botswana. *International Nursing Review, 50*(1), 22-33.

Physicians for Human Rights (PHR). (2004). *An action plan to prevent brain drain. Building equitable health systems in Africa.* Boston, MA: PHR.

Pithouse, R. (2005). Struggle is a school: The rise of a shack dwellers' movement in Durban, South Africa. *Monthly Review, 57*(9).

Poggenpoel, S., & Claasen, M. (2004, December 10). *Budget briefs: No. 150 Provincial Comparative Health Budget Brief 2004.* Institute for Democracy in South Africa. [retrieved on January 4, 2005] Available from: http://www.idasa.org.za/index.asp?page=outputs.asp%3FTID%3D8%260 TID%3D21

Porco, T. (2001). Amplification dynamics: Predicting the effect of HIV on TB outbreaks. *Journal of Acquired Immune Deficiency Syndrome, 28,* 437-444.

Qotole, M. (2001). Worker participation—Now and in the past. In N. Newman, J. Pape, & H. Jansen (Eds.), *Is there an alternative? South African workers confronting globalization.* Cape Town: International Labor Resource and Information Group.

Reilly, P. (2003). Importing controversy; U.S. hospitals' recruitment of foreign nurses stirs debate as poorer countries struggle with staffing shortages of their own. *Modern Healthcare, 33*(13), 20-28.

Republic of South Africa (RSA). (1990). Draft National Policy on Testing for HIV. Department of Health. National Policy for Health Act (Act No. 116 of 1990).

Republic of South Africa (RSA). (1993a). Compensation for Occupational Injuries and Diseases Act (COIDA), Act 130 of 1993 Department of Labour, GG No. 15158.

Republic of South Africa (RSA). (1993b). Hazardous Biological Agents Regulations, Occupational Health and Safety Act (OSHA), Act 85 of 1993 Department of Labour, GG No. 14918.

Republic of South Africa (RSA). (1996). Growth, employment and redistribution, a macroeconomic strategy. Available from: http://www.polity.org.za/html/govdocs/policy/growth.html

Republic of South Africa (RSA). (1996). South Africa Department of Finance. Growth, employment and redistribution, a macroeconomic strategy. [retrieved March 15, 2004] Available from: http://www.polity.org.za/html/govdocs/policy/growth.html

Republic of South Africa (RSA). (1997). White paper on health transformation. South Africa Department of Health. GG No. 17910.

Republic of South Africa (RSA). (1999). Management of Occupational Exposure to the Human Immunodeficiency Virus (HIV). South African Department of Health. HIV/AIDS and STD Directorate1999. [retrieved on December 1, 2004] Available from: http://www.doh.gov.za/search/index.html

Republic of South Africa (RSA). (2000). Code of Good Practice: Key Aspects of HIV/AIDS and Employment, Labour Relations Act, 1995 (Act No. 66 of 1995), Employment Equity Act, 1998 (Act No. 55 of 1998). GG No. 21815.

Republic of South Africa (RSA). (2003a). Operational Plan for Comprehensive HIV and AIDS Care, Management and Treatment for SA. Available from: http://www.gov.za/issues/hiv/careplan19nov03.htm

Republic of South Africa (RSA). (2003b). South African National Treasury. *Intergovernmental Fiscal Review, 2003,* 79. Pretoria, South Africa. Available from: www.tresaury.gov.za

Republic of South Africa (RSA). (2004a). Draft Circular Instruction Regarding Compensation for Occupationally Acquired HIV. No. 183, Government Notice No. 1349, GG, Vol. 473 No. 27003.

Republic of South Africa (RSA). (2004b). South African Department of Health. Public hospitals: A decade of transformation. *Service Delivery Review, 3*(1), 58-64. Available from: http://www.dpsa.gov.za/documents/service_delivery_review/vol3ed1/public%20hospitals.pdf

Republic of South Africa (RSA). (2006). Department of Health Annual Report 2005/2006. [retrieved November 24, 2009] Available from: www.info.gov.za

Rosenberg, T. (2001, January 28). Look at Brazil. *The New York Times, Sunday Magazine.* Sec. 6, p. 26.

Rowden, R. (2004, September). Blocking progress: How the fight against HIV/AIDS is being undermined by the World Bank and International Monetary Fund. A policy briefing by ActionAid International USA, Global AIDS Alliance, Student Global AIDS Campaign, RESULTS Educational Fund.

Rowthorn, R., & Wright, R. (1998). Globalization and economic convergence: An assessment. Discussion paper no. 131, United Nations Conference on Trade and Development. New York: UNCTAD.

Sagoe-Moses, C., Pearson, R., Perry, J., & Jagger, J. (2001). Risks to health care workers in developing countries. *New England Journal of Medicine, 345*(7), 538-541.

Sassen, S. (1990). U.S. immigration policy toward Mexico in a global economy. *Journal of International Affairs, 43*(2), 369-384.

Saul, J. (2001). Cry for the beloved country: A special report on neoliberalism and post-apartheid South Africa. *Monthly Review, 52*(8).

Schneider, H. (2002). On the fault line: The politics of AIDS policy in contemporary South Africa. *African Studies, 61*(1), 145-167.

Schneider, H., & Fassin, D. (2002). Denial and defiance: A socio-political analysis of AIDS in South Africa. *AIDS, 16,* S45-S51.

Schneider, H., & Fassin, D. (2003). The politics of AIDS in South Africa: Beyond the controversies. *British Medical Journal, 326*(7387), 495-497.

Schneider, H., & Stein, J. (2001). Implementing AIDS policy in post-apartheid South Africa. Social Science and Medicine, 52(5), 723-731.

Schoepf, B., Schoepf, C., & Millen, J. (2000). Theoretical therapies, remote remedies: SAPs and the political ecology of poverty and health in Africa. In J. Y. Kim, J. Millen, I. Irwin, & J. Gershman (Eds.), *Dying for growth: Global inequality and the health of the poor.* Monroe, ME: Common Courage Press.

Schwartz, S., Susser, E., & Susser, M. (1999). A future for epidemiology? *Annual Reviews of Public Health, 20,* 15-33.

Shaffer, E., & Brenner, J. (2004). Trade and health care: Corporatizing vital human services. In M. Fort, M. A. Mercer, & O. Gish (Eds.), *Sickness and wealth: The corporate assault on global health* (pp. 79-94). Cambridge, MA: South End Press.

Shaffer, E., Witzkin, H., Brenner, J., & Jasso-Aguila, R. (2005). Global trade and public health. *American Journal of Public Health, 95*(1), 23-34.

Shange, Z. (2002. March). Occupational Health Sister, King Edward VII hospital, Durban. Interview.

Shevel, A. (2003). Hospitals offer incentives in a bid to keep their staff. Health systems trust. Durban: HST, June. [retrieved on March 1, 2004] Available from: http://news. hst.org.za/view.php3?id=20030207

Shisana, O., Hall, E. J., Maluleke, R., Chauveau, J., & Schwabe, C. (2004). HIV/AIDS prevalence among South African health workers. *South African Medical Journal, 94*(10), 846-850.

Slattery, M. (1998). The epidemic hazards of nursing: Nurses lobby for safer workplace conditions. *American Journal of Nursing, 98*(11), 50-53.

Slevin, P. (2003). I know no one who's died of AIDS, says Mbeki. The Mercury, Sept. 26; A1. [retrieved on December 15, 2004] Available from: http://www.journaids. org/reports/26092003c.htm

Sontag, D. (2004). Early tests for U.S. in its global fight on AIDS. *New York Times,* Jul. 14; Sect. A:1 (col. 2).

South African Municipal Workers Union/Rural Development Services Network. (2000). The cholera epidemic in South Africa and the government's attack on the working class. Joint Press Statement October 26th, 3 pm. [retrieved on November 21, 2004] Available from: http://www.labournet.de/internationales/suedafrika/samwu-rdsn.html

South African Nursing Council. (1999). *HIV/AIDS policy.* South African Nursing Council. [retrieved on December 3, 2004] Available from: http://www.sanc.co.za/ policyhiv.htm

South African Nursing Council. (2004). *Geographical distribution of the population of South Africa versus nursing manpower.* [retrieved December 4, 2004] Available from: http://www.sanc.co.za/stats/stat2003/Distribution%202003xls.htm

South African Press Association. (2001). Legislate against HIV stigma urges UNAIDS chief. SAPA Sept 5. [retrieved on October 12, 2004] Available from: http://www. hst.org.za/news/20010904.

Stack, L., & Hlela, K. (2002). *Enhancing policy implementation: Lessons from the health sector. Social policy series, research report 94. Centre for Policy Studies, University of Witwatersrand.* [retrieved on September 7, 2004] Available from: http:// www.cps.org.za/cps%20pdf/RR94.pdf

Stake, R. E. (1995). *The art of case study research.* Thousand Oaks, CA: Sage Publications.

Statistics South Africa. (2001). 2001 census key results. Pretoria: SSA. [retrieved on December 20, 2004] Available from: http://www.statssa.gov.za/census01/HTML/ Key%20results_files/Key%20results.pdf

Statistics South Africa. (2002). Earning and spending in South Africa: Selected findings and comparisons from the income and expenditure surveys of October 1995 and October 2000. Pretoria: SSA. [retrieved on August 20, 2004] Available from: http:// www.statssa.gov.za/Publications/earningspending2000/earningspending2000October 2000.pdf

Statistics South Africa. (2005). Mortality and causes of death in South Africa, 1997-2003: Findings from death notification. Statistical release P0309.3. Pretoria, South Africa. Available from: http://www.hst.org.za/publications/647

Stein, Z., & Zwi, A. (Eds.). (1990). Maputo Statement on HIV and AIDS in Southern Africa. Action on AIDS in Southern Africa. Proceedings of Maputo Conference on

Health in Transition in Southern Africa. April 9-16. CHISA and HIV Center for Clinical and Behavioral Studies, Columbia University.

Susser, I. (2002). Health rights for women in the age of AIDS. *International Journal of Epidemiology, 31*(1), 45-48.

Susser, M. (1999). Pioneering community-oriented primary care. [Historical Article. Journal Article] *Bulletin of the World Health Organization, 77*(5), 436-438.

Tabb, W. (2001). *The amoral elephant: Globalization and the struggle for social justice in the twenty-first century.* New York: Monthly Review Press.

The barefoot doctor fights AIDS. (2003). [editorial] *The New York Times.* Nov. 28; Sect. A:42.

Thom, A. (2003). A losing battle? *Health-e news.* October. [retrieved on October 23, 2004] Available from: http://www.health-e.org.za/news/article.php?uid=20030202.

Treatment Action Campaign (TAC). (2004). General statement from the People's Health Summit, *TAC Newsletter,* July 13. [retrieved on September 11,2004] Available from: http://www.tac.org.za/newsletter/2004/nsI3_07_2004.htm

Turshen, M. (1999). *Privatizing health services in Africa.* New Brunswick, NJ: Rutgers University Press.

Unger, A. (2002). The impact of HIV/AIDS on Health Care Workers in KwaZulu-Natal: The case of the Hlabisa District Hospital. Policy Brief commissioned by HIV/AIDS Education and Research Division (HEARD), University of Natal, Durban for the KwaZulu-Natal Department of Health.

United Nations Department of Economic and Social Affairs (UNDESA). (1986). *Africa's priority programme for economic recovery, 1986-1990.* [retrieved on August 25, 2004] Available from: http://www.un.org/documents/ga/res/spec/aress13-2.htm

United Nations Development Programme (UNDP). (2003). *South Africa Human Development Report 2003. The challenge of sustainable development in South Africa: Unlocking people's creativity.* Oxford: Oxford University Press. Available from: http://www.undp.org.za/NHDRF.htm

United Nations Development Programme (UNDP). (2004). *Human Development Report 2004. Cultural liberty in today's diverse world.* Oxford: Oxford University Press. [retrieved on July 20, 2004] Available from: http://www.undp.org.in/hdr2004/#HDR2004.

United Nations Joint United Nations Programme on HIV/AIDS (UNAIDS). (2004). *World Health Organization (WHO). AIDS epidemic update December.* Geneva: UNAIDS/WHO. [retrieved on January 10, 2005] Available from: http://www.unaids.org/wad2004/EPIupdate2004_html_en/epi04_00_en.htm

UNAIDS: Joint United Nations Programme on HIV/AIDS and World Health Organization (WHO). (2007). AIDS epidemic update. December. Geneva: UNAIDS/WHO. [retrieved on June 12, 2009] Available from http://data.unaids.org/pub/EPISlides/2007/2007_epiupdate_en.pdf

United States Department of Labor. (1996). Recommendations for Workplace Violence Prevention Programs in Late-Night Retail Establishments. Occupational Safety and Health Administration, Washington, DC. Available from: www.osha.gov/Publications/osha3153.html (August 27, 2007).

van Ameringen, M. (1995). Building a new South Africa volume 1. Economic Policy: A Report from the Mission on Economic Analysis and Policy Formulation for post-apartheid South Africa. Ottawa, Canada: International Development Research Center.

Vavi, Z. (2004). A world to win? Perspective on labor and global change. Address by Zwelinzima Vavi, General Secretary, Congress of South African Trade Unions. A conference on global unionism. Inaugural event of the Cornell Global Labor Institute September 23-24. New York City, ILR Conference Center. [retrieved on October 2, 2004] Available from: http://www.ilr.cornell.edu/globallaborinstitute/inaugural Event/index.html

Waitzkin, H. (2003). Report of the WHO commission on macroeconomics and health: A summary and critique. *Lancet, 361,* 523-527.

Watkinson, E., & Makgetla, N. (2002). South Africa's food security crisis. National Labor and Economic Development Institute. Johannesburg: NALEDI. [retrieved on March 18, 2005] Available from: http://www.naledi.org.za

Wilkinson, R. (2002). Income inequality, social cohesion, and health: Clarifying the theory—A reply to Muntaner and Lynch. In V. Navarro (Ed.), *The political economy of social inequalities: Consequences for health and quality of life* (pp. 347-366). Amityville, NY: Baywood.

Willan, S. (2004). Briefing: Recent changes in the South African government's HIV/AIDS policy and its implementation. *African Affairs, 103,* 109-117.

Williams, B. G., & Campbell, C. M. (1996). Mines, migrancy and HIV in South Africa— Managing the epidemic. *South African Medical Journal, 86,* 1249-1251.

Wooding, J., & Levenstein, C. (1999). *The point of production: Work environment in advanced industrial society.* New York: The Guilford Press.

World Bank. (1987). *Financing health services in developing countries: An agenda for reform.* Washington, DC: World Bank.

World Bank. (1993). *World development report: Investing in health 1993.* Oxford: Oxford University Press.

World Health Organization. (1978). Declaration of Alma Ata. International Conference on Primary Health Care, Alma-Ata, USSR, September 6-12, 1978. [retrieved on April 12, 2004] Available from: www.who.int/hprINPH/docs/declaration_almaata.pdf

World Health Organization (WHO). (2003). Strengthening nursing and midwifery: Report by the Secretariat. Fifty-sixth world health assembly, provisional agenda item 14.11.2003; A56/19. [retrieved on January 8, 2003] Available from: http://www.who.int/gb/EB_WHA/PDF/WHA56/ea5619.pdf

World Health Organization (WHO). (2006). Treat, train, retain: The AIDS and health workforce plan. Report on the consultation on AIDS and human resources for health, WHO, Geneva, May 11-12, 2006. Available from: http://www.who.int/hiv/pub/meetingreports/TTRmeetingreport2.pdf

World Trade Organization (WTO). (2001). Declaration on the TRIPS agreement and public health. Doha WTO Ministerial, November 20, 2001. [retrieved on November 15, 2004] Available from: http://www.wto.org/english/thewto_e/minist_e/min01_e/mindecl_trips_e.htm

Yin, R. K. (1994). Case study research: Design and methods. *Applied Social Research Methods Series* (Vol. 5). Thousand Oaks, CA: Sage Publications.

Zierler, S., & Kreiger, N. (1998). HIV infection in women: Social inequalities as determinants of risk. *Critical Public Health, 8*(1), 13-32.

Zwi, A. B., & Cabral, A. (1991). Identifying "high risk situations" for preventing AIDS. *British Medical Journal* (Clinical research ed.), *303*(6816), 1527-1529.

CR SO

Index

Abdool-Karim, Quarraissha, 4-6
Abdool-Karim, Salim, 4-6, 8
Absences, nurse, 101
"Access for All" agenda, 2
Achmat, Zackie, 3
Act-Up, 3, 43
African National Congress (ANC)
    denial of HIV/AIDS as a major social
        problem, 10-11
    failure to respond to HIV/AIDS
        epidemic, 5
    HIV/AIDS treatment plan, approval of
        national, 45
    hospitals, case studies of three public,
        79
    Maputo Statement on HIV/AIDS
        (1990), 9-10, 42
    negotiated peace settlement
        between apartheid government and,
        33-36
    neoliberal policies, hamstrung by,
        151
    nurses critical of, 147
    overseas for jobs, nurses going,
        161-162
    prevention of mother to child
        transmission, 8
    social justice struggles, 163
    White Paper on Health System
        Transformation, 39, 42
African Socialism (Senghor), 21
AIDS Law Project, 43, 45

Alma-Ata Conference (1978), 23-24,
    27, 150
Antiretroviral (ARV) drug combinations
    Brazil and universal access to, 54
    comprehensive health system
        development along with, 159-160
    denial of HIV/AIDS as a major social
        problem, 43
    generics, use of, 7-8, 54
    life expectancy increased by using, 6
    nurses not receiving, 63-64
    pitfalls to the success of public-sector,
        161
    poor people, now acceptable to provide
        treatment for, 55
    post-exposure prophylaxis treatment
        with, 103-104, 106, 122-123,
        136-137
    problems with ARV treatment, 124
    side effects, 104, 122
Apartheid legacy, 34-36
Asia, Southeast, 2-3
Asian Tiger model, 18

Barefoot Doctor program in China, 23
Berg Report (1981), 26
Blood exposure, protocol following,
    105-106, 150
Bond, Patrick, 11
Botswana, 59

Brain drain and health care workers, 2, 3, 12-13, 55-57, 126-127, 152, 161
Brazil, 7, 8, 54
British National Health Service, 23
Bush, George H., 53
Buthelezi, Mangosuthu G., 79

Cameron, Edwin, 45
Caring labor in the formal economy, undervaluing of, 13, 59, 61, 167, 168
Center for Disease Control, U.S. (CDC), 132
Central hospital (CH), 71, 73, 74
    See also Hospitals, case studies of three public; Staffing/occupational health and HIV/AIDS
Chang, Grace, 57
Chen, Lincoln, 2
China, 23, 31
Cholera, 84
Class power and neoliberal globalization, 19
Colonial legacy, 23
Commodification of health care, 12-13, 152
Community and hospitals, linkages between, 142
Community-based mass movements of poor people, 164
Community Oriented Primary Care (COPC), 5, 24
Compensation, workers', 142-143
Confidentiality issues, 85-86, 105, 119, 121, 146
Congress of South African Trade Unions (COSATU), 3, 34, 43, 90, 164-165
Conscientizing, 166
Coovadia, Hoosen, 6, 11
Cornell Global Labor Institute, 164-165
Cost-effectiveness and the value of human life, 6-8, 29, 40
Coworkers, infected, 140
Cuban doctors, 93

Debt crisis, 25-27, 150
Decommodification, 163-164

Denial of HIV/AIDS as a major social problem
    African National Congress, 10-11
    globalization of free market impacting health care, 156-159
    leadership, lack of government, 152-153
    Mbeki, Thabo, 43
    nurses perspectives, 120-121, 146, 150
    underreporting as a consequence of, 125
    Western approaches to health care, distrust of, 45-46
DENOSA, 167
De-skilling of select nursing tasks, 100
Development/health in sub-Saharan Africa, 20-22
Diarrhea, 84
Disability adjusted life years (DALYS), 6
Discrimination against people living with AIDS, 85
Diseases, privatization and increases in, 30
Disinvestment in government health services, 28-29, 151, 158, 160
District hospital (DH), 67-71
    See also Hospitals, case studies of three public; Staffing/occupational health and HIV/AIDS
Dropout rates for public health programs, 65
Durban, 4
    See also individual subject headings
Durban Declaration (2000), 5, 6

Educators, nurses as HIV/AIDS, 141
Elite interests and neoliberal globalization, 19
Environmental Justice Networking Forum, 163

Facing Mount Kenya (Kenyatta), 21
Financial issues and case study of three public hospitals, 81-82
Freedom and Development (Nyerere), 21
Freedom Charter (1955), 33
Free markets. See Neoliberal and Globalization listings
Friedman, Milton, 17

Geiger, Jack, 4, 5, 24
Gender and male/female power differentials, 60, 120-121, 166-168
Gender comparisons of hospital staff and management, 73, 76
General Agreement on Trade in Services (GATS), 162
Generic antiretroviral drug combinations, 7-8, 54
Gini Coefficient, 64
Globalization of free market impacting health care
   African National Congress hamstrung by neoliberal policies, 151
   African policy response to the debt crisis, 26-27
   bad health effects on communities, 15
   debt crisis, 25-27
   denial of HIV/AIDS as a major social problem, 156-159
   health care and development in sub-Saharan Africa, 20-22
   health system development, 22-25
   hospitals, case studies of three public, 154-156
   neoliberalism: ideology or legitimate strategy, 17-20
   privatization's impact on health care delivery, 29
   South Africa and sub-Saharan Africa, 30-32
   structural adjustment policies, 7, 14, 20, 27-29, 150
   See also Neoliberalism in postapartheid South Africa and HIV/AIDS epidemic
Gloves, the use of, 133
Goggles, wearing, 133
Group of 77 (G 77), 22, 24
Growth, Employment and Redistribution (GEAR), 11, 36-38, 46-47

Hani, Chris, 10, 41
Harvard School of Public Health, 7
Hazards faced by service-sector workers
   See also Occupational health and HIV/AIDS; Work environment of nurses

"Health Care in the Americas: A Right or a Luxury" (2004), 1, 3
Health system development in independence era, 22-25
Health Workers for Change Initiative (HWFCI), 59
Heritage Foundation, 27
History of nursing, 50-51
Home-based palliative care, 51
Horizontal integration and primary health care, 24
Hospitals, case studies of three public
   central hospital, 71, 73, 74
   challenges, health care, 77-81
   discussions about HIV/AIDS with patients, nurses refusing to have, 86-87
   district hospital, 67-71
   economy of the communities where they are located, 64-65
   finances, 81-82
   globalization of free market impacting health care, 154-156
   management, hospital, 73, 75-77
   occupational health and HIV/AIDS, 106-116
   policy (healthcare) influenced by political/social conditions, 65-67
   privatization of health care delivery, 66
   regional hospital, 71, 72
   risk of HIV/AIDS, nurses' occupational, 63
   services, impact of HIV/AIDS on, 82-84
   staff, impacts of HIV/AIDS on, 84-87
   summary/conclusions, 149-150
   urban/rural inequalities, 67, 68
   See also Nurses speak; Staffing/occupational health and HIV/AIDS
Human Development Indicators (HDIs), 30-31, 65, 151

Import substitution industrialization (ISI), 21
Indian communities, 146

Indinivir, 104
Individualizing problems at the individual system level, 157-158
Indonesia, 31
Industrial Health Research Group (IHRG), 59, 153-154, 168
Infant mortality rates, 30, 31, 151
Inkatha Freedom Party (IFP), 8, 79
Insurance, self-financing, 29
International AIDS Conference in Durban (2000), 48
International Labor Organization (ILO), 166
International Monetary Fund (IMF)
  borrow billions, African countries encouraged to, 21
  debt crises, 25-26
  decommodification, 164
  negotiated peace settlement between apartheid government and ANC, 36
  neoliberal globalization impacting health care, 18, 20
  structural violence and global disparities of HIV/AIDS, 52
I Speak of Freedom (Nyerere), 21

Joint Learning Initiatives, 56

Kark, Emily, 24, 66
Kark, Sidney, 5, 24, 66
King Edward VIII hospital, 9
KwaZulu-Natal, 4
  See also individual subject headings

Labor/work environment approach to public health, recommendations for a, 169
  See also Work environment of nurses
Lagos Plan of Action (1980), 26
Lamivudine (3TC), 104
Landless People's Movement, 163
Latin America, 21
Legislation
  (South Africa) Compensation for Occupational Injuries and Diseases Act of 1993 (COIDA), 104

Life expectancy, 6, 30
London, Leslie, 4
Lowenson, Rene, 27

Management's control of the workplace and occupational health, 49-50, 73, 75-77, 159
Manuel, Trevor, 35
Maputo Statement on HIV/AIDS (1990), 9-10, 42, 151, 154
Mbeki, Thabo, 10-11, 43, 45
McNeil, Patrick, 8-9
Millennium Development Goals (MDGs), 31-32, 56, 165
Mining industry and social disruption, 34
Moonlighting opportunities for nurses, 91, 102
Morale of health care workers, 8-9
Morality and using cost-effectiveness schedules, 6-7
Mozambique, 25
Municipal Services Project (MSP), 18, 59, 168

National AIDS Convention of South Africa (NACOSA), 42
National Association of People Living with HIV/AIDS (NAPWA), 42
Nationalist movements using democratic principles as rallying points, 21
National Labor and Economic Development Institute (NALEDI), 37-38
Needlestick injuries, 107-109, 111-115, 117-119, 134-136
  See also Nurses speak
Nelson Mandela School of Medicine, 5-6
Neoliberalism in postapartheid South Africa and HIV/AIDS epidemic
  apartheid legacy, 34-36
  Growth, Employment and Redistribution, 36-38
  health care transformation, 38-41

[Neoliberalism in postapartheid South
Africa and HIV/AIDS epidemic]
HIV/AIDS, the explosion of, 41-46
negotiated peace settlement between
apartheid government and ANC,
33-36
summary/conclusions, 46-47
See also Globalization of free market
impacting health care
Netcare, 89
Neviripine, 8, 43, 65, 83
New International Economic Order
(NIEO), 24, 27
Not Yet Uhuru (Odinga), 21
Nurses speak
accidental exposures: how do they
occur?, 134-135
causes of HIV/AIDS, government's
messages about the, 144
community and hospitals, linkages
between, 142
confidentiality issues,
146
contradictory statements made by
nurses, 145
coworkers, infected, 140
denial of having HIV/AIDS, 120-121,
146, 150
educators, nurses as HIV/AIDS,
141
exposure to HIV/AIDS, 131-132
gender dynamics of occupational risk
to HIV/AIDS, 167-168
government not concerned with their
health, 146-147
government policy at the workplace,
142-144
HIV/AIDS policy, critical of
government's, 147
increases in HIV/AIDS and TB
patients, 139-140
Indian communities, 146
interview results summary, group,
171-174
limitations specific to nurse group
interviews, 129-130
management's attitudes, 159

[Nurses speak]
overseas, going, 143-144
overview, 130-131
policy, criticisms of occupational
health, 144
post-exposure prophylaxis, 136-137
precautions and protective policies,
universal, 132-134
relationship between nurses and
patients, 140-141, 147
reporting injuries and filling out forms,
135-136
salaries, 143-144, 147
secrecy, tired of all the, 146, 159
shortage, nursing, 147
suggestions for safer work environment, 144-145
summary/conclusions, 148
treating all patients as positive for
HIV/AIDS, 134
variation of nurses' views, 148,
149
voluntary counseling and testing,
136-137
Nyerere, Julius K., 22

Occupational health and HIV/AIDS
blood exposure, protocol following,
105-106
changes needed, 162-163
confidentiality issues, 105
cost (high) of treatment for HIV
infected nurses, 124-125
denial of HIV/AIDS as a major social
problem, 120-121
failure of the system to protect nurses,
123
hospitals, case studies of three public,
106-116
needlestick injuries, 107-109, 111-115,
117-119
organizing around, 168-169
overview, 102-103
policy on workplace exposure to
HIV/AIDS, 103
post-exposure prophylaxis, 103-104

[Occupational health and HIV/AIDS]
precautions, universal, 105
prevalence of HIV/AIDS among
nurses, 123-124
reporting exposures, nurses not,
118-119
summary/conclusions, 125-127
tuberculosis, HIV infected nurses'
exposure to, 124
voluntary counseling and testing,
nurses' refusing, 121-122
See also Hospitals, case studies of three
public; Nurses speak; Staffing/
occupational health and HIV/AIDS;
Work environment of nurses
Occupational Safety and Health
Administration (OSHA), 50
Oil crises of 1970s, 25
Organization of African Unity (OAU),
22, 26
Overseas for jobs, nurses going, 95-96,
143-144, 152, 161-162

Partners in Health, 7
Pharmaceutical companies and profits
from AIDS medicines, 54
Physicians for Human Rights (PHR), 2
Political/economic forces determining
how health care is delivered, 15
See also Hospitals, case studies of three
public
Political/social/industry context deter-
mining occupational illness, 49-51,
142-144
Post-exposure prophylaxis (PEP),
103-104, 106, 122-123, 136-137
Poverty as a cause of poor health, 30
Power differentials between men and
women, 60, 120-121, 166-168
Precautions, universal, 105, 132-134
President's Emergency Plan for AIDS
Relief (PEPFAR), 53
Prevention of mother to child
transmission (PMTCT), 8, 43,
65, 83

Primary health care (PHC), 23-25, 27, 34,
38, 149, 150-151
Privatization of health care delivery,
28, 29-30, 39-40, 59, 61, 66, 152,
158
Public Health Service, U.S. (PHS), 104
Public-sector universal treatment program
in Brazil, 7, 8, 54

Racial composition of hospital staff and
management, 73, 76
Reconstruction and Development
Programme (RDP), 36-38
Recruiting nurses, 96-98
Regional hospital (RH), 71, 72
See also Hospitals, case studies of three
public; Staffing/occupational health
and HIV/AIDS
Reporting injuries and filling out forms,
nurses' views on, 118-119, 125,
135-136
Research on nurses/HIV-AIDS/occupa-
tional health, 57-61
Retirees, rehiring, 99-100
Risk behavior vs. social inequality and
HIV/AIDS epidemic, 52-53
Rockefeller Foundation, 158

Salaries for nurses, 94-95, 143-144, 147,
150, 161, 167
Saudi Arabia, 94-96
Selective strategies, 27, 151
Service-sector workers, analyzing hazards
faced by, 50
Shack-dwellers movement (Abahlali
baseMjondolo), 164
Shortage, nursing, 2-3, 55-57, 90-94,
100, 102, 126-127, 147, 161-162
Simelala, Nono, 123
Social inequalities and the HIV/AIDS
epidemic, 10, 52-53, 60, 120-121,
125, 152, 158, 166-167

Social movements influencing spread/
treatment of HIV/AIDS, 8, 54,
163-168
Social Unionism, 13
South Africa
Community Oriented Primary Care, 24
devastating impact from HIV/AIDS,
why has South Africa suffered this,
51-55
Freedom Charter, 33
home-based palliative care, 51
human development indicators,
30-31
Millennium Development Goals,
31-32
prevalence of HIV/AIDS, 5, 10, 34,
41, 43, 83
treatment and care plan releases in
2003, 160-161
See also African National Congress
(ANC); individual subject headings
South Africa Municipal Workers Union
(SAMWU), 59, 168
South African Communist Party (SACP),
34
Southern African Migration Project
(SAMP), 53
Soviet Union, collapse of the, 35, 156
Soweto Electricity Crisis Committee,
163
Staffing/occupational health and
HIV/AIDS
absences, nurse, 101
background, staffing, 89-90
background on occupational health
and safety, 90
moonlighting to supplement wages,
91, 102
overseas exodus, 95-96
policymaking/implementation, nurses'
lack of involvement in, 13, 14, 150,
165-166
problems for nurses similar in world
class and deprived hospitals, 126
recruiting nurses, 96-98
retirees, rehiring, 99-100
salaries, 94-95

[Staffing/occupational health and
HIV/AIDS]
shortage dynamics, hospital-level,
90-94, 100, 102
threats that health care workers face in
developing countries, 14
work organization changes to cope
with nurse shortages, 100
See also Nurses speak; Occupational
health and HIV/AIDS; Work
environment of nurses
Stein, Mervyn, 4-5
Stein, Zena, 4-5
Stigma attached to having HIV/AIDS, 48,
85, 121, 125, 146, 150, 152-153,
156-159, 168
Strategies for Social Justice Movements
from Southern Africa to the United
States (Bond), 163
Structural adjustment policies (SAPs), 7,
14, 20, 27-29, 150
Structural violence and global disparities
of HIV/AIDS, 52

Tanzania, 23-24
Testing nursing for HIV/AIDS, 9
See also Voluntary counseling and
testing
Toxicity of AIDS drugs, 122
Treatment Action Campaign (TAC), 3,
42, 43-45, 153, 163
Treatment Action Group (TAG), 3, 6
TRIPS agreement under the World Trade
Organization, 43, 54
Trucking routes and the spread of
HIV/AIDS, 53
Tuberculosis (TB), 83-84, 124, 139-140

Unions, trade
"A World to Win," 164-165
background on occupational health and
safety, 90
occupational health policy and black,
disconnect between, 61
perspective on HIV/AIDS policy, 3
social unionism, 13
struggle for HIV/AIDS treatment, 43

[Unions, trade]
  white craft-based, 90
  women not getting appropriate help
    from, 167-168
United Democratic Front (UDF), 34
United Kingdom, 95
United Nations, 26
  Conference for Trade and Development
    (UNCTAD), 22
  Development Program, 30-31
  UNICEF, 27
United States, characteristics of work
  environment in, 12-13
United States Aid for International
  Development (USAID), 27
United States and Human Development
  Index, 31
Universal public-sector program for
  HIV/AIDS treatment, value of,
  160-161
Universal treatment program in Brazil,
  public-sector, 7, 8, 54
University of Cape Town (UCT), 153,
  168
University of Natal, 5-6
Urban/rural inequalities in healthcare
  services, 67, 68
User fees, 29

Vavi, Zwelinzima, 164-165
Voices of health care workers, listening
  to, 13, 14
Voluntary counseling and testing
  (VCT), 64, 105-106, 121-122,
  136-137
Vulnerability of workforce, cheap
  labor/deregulation and the, 50-51
  See also Occupational health and
    HIV/AIDS; Work environment of
    nurses

Western approaches to health care,
  distrust of, 45-46
White Paper on Health System
  Transformation (1997), 39, 42,
  149

"Who Cares for Health Care Workers?",
  59, 61, 168
Without Bitterness (Orizu), 21
Women's burdens and the HIV/AIDS
  epidemic, 60, 120-121
Work environment of nurses
  history of nursing, 50-51
  political/economic forces deter-
    mining how health care is delivered,
    15
  political/social/industry context
    determining occupational illness,
    49-51
  recommendations for a labor/work
    environment approach to public
    health, 169
  research on nurses/HIV-AIDS/occupa-
    tional health, 57-61
  shortage of nurses, brain drain and the,
    55-57
  theory of the work environment,
    49-51
  United States, characteristics of work
    environment in, 12-13
  well being of workforce attached to
    health of patients, 13-14
  See also Hospitals, case studies of
    three public; Nurses speak; Occu-
    pational health and HIV/AIDS;
    Staffing/occupational health and
    HIV/AIDS
World Bank
  borrow billions, African countries
    encouraged to, 21
  debt crises, 25-26
  decommodification, 164
  Growth, Employment and
    Redistribution, 37
  neoliberal globalization impacting
    health care, 18, 20
  selective strategies, 27
  shortage, nursing, 56
  structural adjustment policies,
    28
World Health Organization (WHO),
  19-20, 23, 57, 59

World Organization for the Right to
    Health Care, Inc. (WORPHC), 1
World Trade Organization (WTO), 18,
    43, 54, 164
Wretched of the Earth, The (Fanon),
    21

Xhosa people, 79

Zambia, 25
Zidovudine (AZT), 103-104
Zimbabwe, 23, 24-25, 151
Zulu people, 79

A SELECTION OF TITLES FROM THE

WORK, HEALTH AND ENVIRONMENT SERIES

Series Editors, *Charles Levenstein, Robert Forrant and John Wooding*

AT THE POINT OF PRODUCTION
The Social Analysis of Occupational
and Environmental Health
Edited by Charles Levenstein

BEYOND CHILD'S PLAY
Sustainable Product Design in the
Global Doll-Making Industry
Sally Edwards

ENVIRONMENTAL UNIONS
Labor and the Superfund
Craig Slatin

METAL FATIGUE
American Bosch and the Demise
of Metalworking in the Connecticut River Valley
Robert Forrant

SHOES, GLUES AND HOMEWORK
Dangerous Work in the Global Footwear Industry
Pia Markkanen

WITHIN REACH?
Managing Chemical Risks in Small Enterprises
David Walters

INSIDE AND OUT
Universities and Education for Sustainable Development
Edited by Robert Forrant and Linda Silka

WORKING DISASTERS
The Politics of Recognition and Response
Edited by Eric Tucker

LABOR-ENVIRONMENTAL COALITIONS
Lessons from a Louisiana Petrochemical Region
Thomas Estabrook

CORPORATE SOCIAL RESPONSIBILITY
FAILURES IN THE OIL INDUSTRY
Edited by Charles Woolfson and Matthias Beck